Super Healthy Hair, Skin and Nails

By the same author:

Easy Pregnancy with Yoga
Pain-free Periods
Secrets of Stopping Hair Loss
Super Natural Immune Power

Super Healthy Hair, Skin and Nails

Stella Weller

Illustrated by Bee Walters

Thorsons
An Imprint of HarperCollins*Publishers*

Thorsons
An Imprint of HarperCollins*Publishers*
77-85 Fulham Palace Road,
Hammersmith, London W6 8JB

First published by Thorsons 1988
Revised edition published 1991
1   3   5   7   9   10   8   6   4   2

A catalogue record for this book
is available from the British Library

ISBN 0 7225 2596 6

Typeset by Harper Phototypesetters Limited,
Northampton, England
Printed in Great Britain by
HarperCollinsManufacturing, Glasgow

CONTENTS

I thank everyone who has helped me prepare this book by providing encouragement and useful information.

I am particularly grateful to Carol Beaumont, John Hardaker, Dr David Horrobin, Maxwell Noble, Brenda Reynolds, Lucyna Sloane, the staff of Surrey Centennial Library (Guildford, Canada), Bee Walters, and Walter Weller.

LIST OF ILLUSTRATIONS

INTRODUCTION

Hair, skin and nails are among the most visible parts of our body. Because we can see and touch them, they play an important part in shaping our self-image. Their condition and appearance substantially affect how we feel, how we regard ourselves and how we function.

Hair, skin and nails are those parts of us our friends, relatives and acquaintances see. How they look partially determines to what extent we are able to socialize comfortably. They influence how confident we feel. And although few hair, skin and nail disorders are entirely a result of our emotions, there are virtually none that do not profoundly affect our feelings.

We've finally acknowledged that skin is not merely a means of protection for vital structures but itself a major one. It is in fact our largest organ, representing about 15 per cent of our body weight.

Although skin is on the outside of the body and on view, its care is not only an external affair but an internal matter as well. Informed, intelligent health consumers and professionals therefore take an inside-outward as well as an outside-inward approach to looking after it.

Like other body tissues, skin requires nourishment from within to stay healthy and repair itself when damaged. All nutrients taken in through a wholesome diet work together to this end, but there are some which experts consider especially important to the integrity and attractiveness of skin, and to that of hair and nails, which are really modified forms of skin. Among these are special substances vital to the billions of cells that make up skin tissue, and to the natural lubricant that keeps it and the hair resilient. These nutrients are also essential for strong, healthy nails.

Although skin is waterproof, some products are readily absorbed through its tiny openings, thus providing an external complement to the dietary factors supplied internally. Together, they represent total nutrition for this major organ.

Skin, hair and nails are reliable indicators of our general state of health, and perhaps nowhere else in the body do deficiencies manifest themselves so vividly.

Happily, however, the rewards of intelligent nutrition — from within and from without — regular, appropriate exercise and relaxation, and the discriminating use of natural skin, hair and nail care products are equally apparent.

This book throws light on all these aspects of care which are crucial to the health and attractiveness of the skin, hair and nails. And because the key to looking after these structures wisely is understanding how they are put together and what their functions are, I have included a chapter that provides the necessary background information (see Chapter 1).

I have also discussed deviations from the normal condition of the skin, hair and nails and what these could mean. While most are not life threatening, they can make our existence uncomfortable.

Included, too, are the effects of stress, smoking, alcohol, medications and sun on the skin and hair, and practical measures for dealing with these.

Skin specialists and cosmetic experts are seeing, and will continue to see, more and more individuals with skin, hair and nail disorders. Although many of these problems are of minimal medical importance, they represent a major cosmetic concern for the person experiencing them.

As people become increasingly aware and knowledgeable about health and health disorders, they are taking more responsibility for their bodies. They are also placing greater emphasis on self-image. These trends have led to a heightened interest in safe, effective self-treatment.

I believe that the contents of this book will provide you with the information necessary to plan and carry out the type of care that will bring forth qualities characteristic of superb health: strong nails, lustrous hair and firm, problem-free skin.

1. UNDERSTANDING YOUR HAIR, SKIN AND NAILS

The key to looking after your hair, skin and nails intelligently is understanding how they are constructed and what their functions are. It is only when you are equipped with this information that you can sensibly plan and carry out the type of care that will bring out those qualities that are unmistakable signs of healthy hair, skin and nails.

An acquaintance with the structure and function of these tissues is therefore of value. I do believe that even if you read through this chapter only once, you will benefit from it as you embark on what will perhaps turn out to be the wisest approach you have yet taken toward acquiring and maintaining optimum health and attractiveness of these most visible parts of your body.

Skin

More than just a covering
Your skin is more than just an integument, or external covering, for your body. It is an essential organ — the largest and one of the most important that you own, making up about 15 per cent of your body weight. You have about 21 square feet (approximately 2 square metres) of skin. In only 1 square inch of it (about 6 square centimetres), there are 650 sweat glands, about 20 blood vessels, 78 heat receptors, 13 cold receptors, 1,300 nerve endings to record pain, 19,500 sensory cells at the ends of nerve fibres, about 165 touch receptors, 100 sebaceous glands, 65 hairs and muscles and a total of about 19,500,000 cells.

The well-known American dermatologist Irwin Lubowe (see Bibliography) has described the skin as a busy message centre, more complicated than the best man-made electronic brain. By way of its nerve endings, it rapidly transmits sensations of heat, cold, pain and danger to the brain and relays responses to the muscles, which then respond by reflex action.

Skin is a metabolically active boundary between you and your environment. Pliable yet tough, it is your natural armour, cushioning deeper organs and protecting the entire body against heat and cold, external injuries such as bumps, cuts and damage from chemicals, as well as shielding against the entry of bacteria ('germs') that live on its surface by means of an 'acid mantle'.

Exciting similarities have been found between the epithelial cells of the skin and those of the thymus gland, an important immune system structure. These discoveries offer compelling evidence in favour of skin being an integral part of the immune system, our chief resource for defending against damage from harmful agents. (For fuller information on the role of skin in immunity, do read my book entitled *Super Natural Immune Power*, details of which are given in the Bibliography.)

The skin's surface is never sterile. It is colonized by flora (literally plant life) which includes a variety of 'germs'. There is considerable evidence that, far from being harmful, these resident 'germs' actually discourage the growth on the skin of more powerful organisms. More potent, though, is the skin's upper-most, cornified layer, coated with a fluid lipid (fat) film which contains unsaturated fatty acids (see Chapter 2). This film has an important bactericidal action, that is, it has the ability to destroy harmful germs.

This uppermost skin layer helps to control water loss and so prevent dehydration. Yet, although waterproof, there are openings — pores — which permit the absorption of oxygen and certain substances that may be applied to the skin, such as creams, lotions, oils, and so on. The skin is, in effect, a reservoir for nutrients.

In addition, the skin may be considered a minor excretory system, helping to eliminate salts, water and urea (the final product of protein metabolism) in the perspiration.

As a secretory organ, the skin releases sebum, the fatty product of the sebaceous, or oil-secreting, glands, which is the body's natural lubricant.

Yet another function of the skin — one of the most intriguing — is pigmentation, or colouring. Cells in the skin's basal layer convert a protein building-block (amino acid) into the pigment known as melanin. For skin not protected by hair or clothing, melanin is the only substantial means of defence against the sun's damaging ultraviolet light (see also Chapter 9). Without melanin, the epidermis (the outer portion of the skin) is little more than a thin, transparent membrane which is practically useless as protection against ultraviolet radiation. The skin synthesizes vitamin D through the action of sunlight on the modified cholesterol molecules it contains.

As a temperature regulator, skin aids in both the loss and retention of heat. Body temperature is fairly constant in healthy humans. It is maintained by an adjustment between heat production and heat loss and these are controlled by heat regulation centres in the hypothalamus, located in the brain. It is through the sweat glands and blood circulatory system that this balance is maintained. Eighty-five per cent of body heat is lost through the skin.

When skin is exposed to heat or when the internal temperature of the body begins to rise, the small arteries (blood vessels) of the skin dilate, or widen, to allow more blood to flow through them so as to promote heat loss. Conversely, when the skin is exposed to cold or when the body's internal temperature begins to drop, the blood vessels constrict, or tighten, to impede blood flow through them. Thus, less heat is lost from the body.

Finally, the skin may be regarded as a medium of expression. It can speak eloquently of feelings such as embarrassment through blushing; of anger through redness; of fear through paleness and of anxiety through sweating.

Skin structure
The skin is a structural marvel. Essentially, it is composed of two

layers: the *epidermis*, or cuticle, and the *dermis*, or corium.

The epidermis — the outer part — is a mosaic made up of four main layers of *stratified epithelium*, so called because it consists of more than one stratum, or horizontal layer of cells. It varies in depth from less than 0.1 millimetre on the eyelids to more than 1 millimetre on the soles of the feet.

The outermost of these layers — the *stratum corneum* — is formed of several layers of flattened cells which have lost their nuclei and become horn-like, and which contain *keratin*, an exceedingly tough protein substance. Keratin has waterproofing properties and so prevents water loss from deeper tissues. It is also found in hair and nails.

The *stratum corneum* gives protection to body surfaces from extremes of temperature and external injuries. It is most delicate on the eyelids and toughest on the soles and palms.

Directly below is the *stratum lucidum* which, as the name suggests, is a clear layer formed of flattened, translucent cells.

Beneath is the *stratum granulosum* which consists of two or three layers of flattened cells containing granules of *eleidin*, a precursor, or forerunner, of keratin.

The final layer of epidermis is known as the *stratum germinativum*, composed of two layers of well-formed epithelial cells: *prickle cells*, so named because the minute fibrils that connect one cell to another give a prickly appearance, and *basal cells*, from which new epidermal cells are constantly being produced.

There is continuous movement and change in each of these skin layers. As the cells of the outer layer become hard and lose their nuclei, they are shed and replaced by new ones which migrate upward. This process is called *keratinization*. It usually takes about 15 days, or 360 hours, when we're younger, and slows down as we become older. But it doesn't stop. Thus, the skin's wonderful properties of self-renewal mean that we have a fresh chance, every day, to be healthier and more attractive.

The dermis, which may be likened to the foundation of a building, is composed of dense fibrous and elastic connective tissue. It is divided into two layers.

The superficial *papillary layer* has cone-like projections which fit into corresponding depressions in the epidermis above. These result in fingerprints. The blood supply in this layer is rich. It provides nutrients for the epidermis and allows heat to radiate to the skin surface. It is here, too, that pain and tactile (touch) receptors are located.

The deep *reticular layer* houses blood vessels, oil and sweat glands, hair follicles and pressure receptors. It is composed mainly of white fibrous tissue supporting the structures it contains.

Throughout the dermis, *collagen* and *elastic fibres* are found. The former is responsible for the toughness of the skin and the latter gives it its elasticity, making it 'young'. As we age, the number of elastic fibres decreases and the subcutaneous (under the skin) tissue loses fat. The skin consequently becomes less resilient, wrinkles and sags.

Although not considered part of the skin, the subcutaneous tissue is related to it and serves two useful functions: it acts as a shock absorber, and it insulates the deeper tissues from the effects of extreme changes in temperature outside the body.

Cutaneous glands

The cutaneous (skin) glands fall into two groups:

Sebaceous glands are found all over the skin, except on the soles and in the palms. They are called *exocrine glands*. Some of their ducts open directly onto the skin surface; most empty into hair follicles.

The *sudoriferous glands* (sweat glands) secrete perspiration through pores in the skin. An adult has about two million sweat glands and can produce about one litre of sweat per day, but this amount varies with muscular activity and atmospheric conditions.

There are two types of sudoriferous glands: *eccrine* and *apocrine*. The former are found all over the body and produce clear perspiration. The latter are largely found in the axillae (armpits) and genital area. They secrete a milky substance containing proteins, as well as the substances found in eccrine secretions.

Sweat glands are most numerous in the palms of the hands and soles of the feet. They are an important part of the body's heat-regulating equipment.

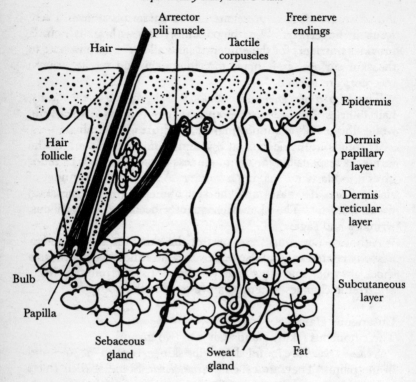

Figure 1: Diagram of skin section and underlying tissues

Bloody supply to the skin

The blood vessels supplying the skin are so numerous that they can hold a large proportion of the body's entire blood supply. This is very important indeed to the nourishment of the billions of cells skin tissue contains.

Interference with the skin's blood supply causes cells to die and ulcerated areas to appear. An example of this is seen in patients confined to bed and those who lie in one position for too long. The body's weight exerts pressure on the skin, especially over bony parts, and reduces blood flow to the tissues. Bedsores develop in these areas.

The worst bedsore I've yet seen had penetrated so deeply that the bone was visible. When the patient's nutrition was improved, her position changed frequently and healing agents applied to the skin itself, the diseased area improved remarkably in a few weeks.

Nerve supply to the skin

The skin is generously supplied with nerve fibres of different types. These carry impulses to and from the central nervous system, and it is by means of this arrangement that we acquire information about the world in our immediate vicinity and react appropriately.

Touch, pressure, heat, cold and pain receptors in the skin and underlying tissues comprise what are known as the cutaneous (skin) senses. The number of each type varies: heat receptors are the least numerous. Pain receptors are the most abundant and it is estimated that there are several million scattered throughout the body.

Hair

Hair is often referred to as an appendage of the skin, a supplementary part if you like. The word suggests an afterthought and yet, hair is more than something affixed to the body. It is attached to a truly living, reproducing structure — the so-called root, which is located beneath the surface of the scalp. Within this root are living cells. These produce hair.

Hair is thus an integral part of your body, thriving in health and languishing in illness. In fact, doctors can find clues as to what is taking place in your body by examining your hair.

Functions

Hair has important functions. Although no one will contest that a healthy head of hair is a potent agent of sexual attraction, hair is not simply an adornment. It is one of the body's important protectors from external damage, acting as a solar screen and helping to guard the skull from minor injuries. It keeps the head warm and acts as a valuable sensory structure.

The scalp
Scalp includes skin, the structure and functions of which have already been described. It also comprises dense subcutaneous tissue, *occipito-frontalis muscle* which extends from the back of the head and over it to the eyebrows, *galea*, which is a flattened, tendon-like structure, underlying tissue and *cranial periosteum*, which is fibrous membrane covering the skull, or cranium. This membrane provides support for blood vessels and tendons, protects the bones of the skull and helps in their repair following injury.

Even in cases where much hair has been lost and the scalp seems smooth, there are countless minute openings: pores for the excretion of sweat; follicles for the hair shafts and openings of the sebaceous glands.

The papillae
Beneath each hair shaft is a *papilla* (Latin for 'nipple'; plural, 'papillae'). This is the hair's manufacturing plant in effect. The base of each hair widens and fits snugly into the projection of the papilla. The papilla contains tiny blood vessels, or capillaries, which are part of the blood circulatory system providing nutrients to all tissues.

Anatomy of a hair
Starting at the bottom, a single hair emerges from a papilla and tapers upward from its bulb.

Under a microscope, the circumference of your hair will appear round if your hair is straight. If it is wavy it will look oval and if curly it will appear flat.

The bulb of the hair follicle is divided into a lower and an upper part. The lower part is composed of mitotic, or dividing, cells. The upper part contains cells responsible for producing the inner hair sheath and the hair shaft.

Splitting hairs
A single hair strand is actually thick enough to be divided into three layers, not unlike the layers of the skin's stratified epi-

thelium. Hair is, in fact, modified epithelium.)

The outermost, or horny, layer is called the *cuticle*. It is the sturdy, hardened layer of the hair shaft. It is composed of countless tiny scales, called *imbrications*, which overlap — like the shingles on a rooftop — and are hinged to open or close.

The middle layer — the *cortex* — is composed of elastic material which gives the hair resilience and flexibility. This layer contains the hair's colouring matter. The innermost layer — the *medulla* — may be compared to bone marrow. It is through the medulla that hair absorbs its nourishment.

The molecules of each layer of hair are laced together in seven coiled strands. Scientists believe that these strands are held firmly together by a constant supply of protein.

Hair muscles

You've undoubtedly heard the saying about hair 'standing on end' and you can take it literally. For attached to the hair shafts are tiny muscles called the *arrector pili* muscles which cause the hairs to be erect, as their name suggests.

Under nervous influence, these muscles contract, causing the hairs to which they're attached to become rigid. The goose bumps you get are a result of the arrector pili muscles in action. Here, we have a glimpse of how the state of the nervous sytem can affect the condition of the hair.

Hair growth cycle

Hair grows, on average, about 0.35 millimetre a day, that is about $1/_{72}$ inch, or 1 inch (2.5 centimetres) every two and a half months. It has a long growth period called the *anagen* stage, and this usually lasts between two and six years. There is a short rest period, or *telogen* stage of about three months, and in between these two a *catagen* stage which is a period of transition.

At any given time, about 85 per cent of hair is in the growing stage and 15 per cent is in the resting stage. During the latter, hair is gradually being shed. Normal daily hair loss is between 20 and 100 hairs. Summer heat increases the rate of hair growth but ultraviolet rays do not.

As we age , the rate of hair loss tends to exceed its rate of new growth. We have to lose about 40 per cent of our hair, though, before thinning becomes blatantly obvious.

Nails

Nails are horn-like structures produced by the epidermis. They are usually taken for granted until their function is lost.

Nail functions

Nails protect the distal (end) portion of fingers and toes. They enhance our sense of touch and enable us to pick up small objects. These functions may be adversely affected by a number of factors: infection, changes associated with some skin disorders, medical conditions and tumours, to name a few.

Nail structure

The *nail plate*, the hard, visible part, is a complex protein structure. It grows from the *nail matrix*, located underneath and behind the *lunula* (Latin for 'little moon'), which is the white part from which the nail grows forward.

The matrix is composed of living cells which work together to produce the nail plate. You may find it useful to think of the matrix as the nails' manufacturing plant. Most of the matrix is hidden by the skin proximal to the nail plate (nearest the body) but its most distal portion can be seen through the nail as the pale, half-moon-shaped lunula.

The nail plate is firmly attached to the *nail bed*, which is the skin under the nail itself. The nail plate is surrounded on three sides by *nail folds* and the skin growing onto the nail from the nail folds is the *cuticle*, a delicate and important structure, about which more information is given in Chapter 10.

Nail growth

Fingernails grow between 1 and 2 millimetres a week, which means that it takes about 3 months for a bit of newly manu-

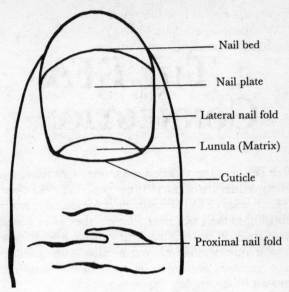

Figure 2: Structure of a nail

factured nail to reach the fingertip. Toenails grow at about half the rate of fingernails, taking about 6 months from matrix to the tip of the toe.

In temperate climates, nails, like hair, tend to grow faster in summer because of increased warmth. In middle and older age, because the matrix usually doesn't make nail as fast as in youth, growth tends to be slower.

Nail growth is also affected by disease and hormone deficiencies. Persistent trauma, such as incurred through nail biting or some forms of stress, can almost double the rate of nail growth. This is a compensatory mechanism whereby epithelium becomes overactive in response to injury or mechanical stress.

2. THE EFA CONNECTION

Over three decades ago, Adelle Davis, one of America's leading nutritionists remarked that, in her opinion, deficiencies of essential fatty acids (EFAs) were more common than realized. In fact, according to the cases she had seen, they were widespread. Now, more than 30 years later, a practising British doctor has made similar observations in connnection with problems that beset large numbers of women in many of the world's affluent countries (see Bibliography: Shreeve).

EFAs and skin
EFAs are a vital part of the structure of every cell in the body. If you consider that in only 1 square inch (about 6 square centimetres) of human skin there are almost 20,000,000 cells, you will need no persuasion to appreciate how crucial EFAs are to the health and attractiveness of the skin, and of the hair and nails which are modified forms of skin.

EFAs are also a necessary component of the fluid lipid (fat) film coating the skin's surface. This film is important for protection against the entry of disease-causing organisms.

When EFAs are a regular part of the diet, they are present in the skin where they act as a sort of antenna. They absorb sunlight into the body and can store this energy for future use in vital biochemical reactions (see Bibliography: Erasmus).

Interestingly, cancer sufferers, who often lack these EFAs in their skin, are allergic to the sun and become easily sunburned.

Fat facts
Before further discussing EFAs, it would be useful to review some

facts about fats themselves, and to become re-acquainted with certain related terms that will appear from time to time in this book.

Fats are needed to provide energy, conserve heat, produce hormones and to help all cells function normally. Any fat can supply calories, but only certain types can fulfil the foregoing vital requirements.

When fats are eaten, they are broken down, during digestion, into glycerin (glycerol) and fatty acids.

Saturated and unsaturated

Fatty acids are often referred to as chains. Adelle Davis has likened them to a charm bracelet containing 'links' for the attachment of 'charms'. Unfilled links, or *unsaturated fatty acids*, allow for the attachment and transportation of nutrients that build cell structure.

Saturated fats. Saturated literally means 'holding all that can be absorbed, received or combined'. Saturated fats tend to raise the cholesterol concentration in the blood. Some even contain cholesterol. These fats are mainly of animal origin (e.g., whole dairy products, lard, meat) and are so constituted chemically as to be incapable of absorbing additional hydrogen.

Polyunsaturated fats. These assist the body in eliminating newly formed cholesterol. They therefore help reduce cholesterol build-up in the walls of arteries (main blood vessels) and keep the level of cholesterol in the blood-stream within normal limits.

Monounsaturated fats. Formerly thought to have no effect on the health of the heart and blood vessels, monounsaturated fats are now believed to help reduce the build-up of fatty deposits in arteries. In the Mediterranean region, for example, where olive and linseed oils are primary sources of dietary fat, the incidence of heart disease is low.

About cholesterol

You may have been wondering why there's so much reference to cholesterol in a book about the health of the hair, skin and nails. Here are the reasons.

Cholesterol is a fat-like material found in many places in the body, for example, in nerve tissue and in the blood. Our bodies do need it — for metabolic purposes, for instance — but too much is undesirable. The surplus tends to stick to the inner walls of blood vessels and this could result in a build-up of fatty and other deposits within the vessels, making them thick and hard, reducing their elasticity and narrowing the passage through which blood has to flow to transport nutrients to all parts of the body.

Every cell depends on an adequate blood supply for its nourishment. In a mere square inch of skin (about 6 square centimetres) there are about 20 blood vessels. Each of us has almost 21 square feet (2 square metres) of skin. If you calculate the number of blood vessels servicing this major organ and consider the consequences if the diameter of each of these blood vessels is substantially reduced, you will appreciate why cholesterol build-up is so detrimental and why, indeed, there has been so much mention of it.

What are essential fatty acids?

Even if we don't eat fats, the body can make some from sugar. There are others, though, that it cannot synthesize and these are called essential fatty acids, or EFAs. They may be likened to vitamins and are in fact sometimes referred to as vitamin F. They were discovered in 1929–30 at the University of Minnesota, USA, by George and Mildred Burr.

EFAs are essential because the body must have them to carry out certain vital functions, yet cannot manufacture them. They have to be furnished by the diet and as such can be considered dietary factors. They are termed essential, too, because their absence creates specific deficiency diseases. One example is a type of eczema in infants caused by a lack in the diet of an essential fatty acid (EFA) called *linoleic acid* (LA).

For years, three fatty acids were considered essential: linoleic, linolenic and arachidonic acids. More recent research has, however, indicated that only linoleic and linolenic (LNA) acids may be so regarded.

Arachidonic acid can be synthesized by the body from LA

provided that vitamin B_6 (pyridoxine) is present. When LNA is undersupplied by the diet, however, serious problems can arise. These include growth retardation, impaired vision, learning disability, lack of motor co-ordination, tingling in the arms and legs and behavioural changes. All these symptoms can be cleared up when LNA is added to the diet.

Functions of EFAs
EFAs are important because:
(1) they are constituents of all membranes in all tissues in the body. For this reason, it should be no surprise that when they are undersupplied, disturbances occur in *all* body tissues.
(2) they are building-blocks from which a group of short-lived molecules called prostaglandins (PGs) are made. In other words, they are precursors, or forerunners, of PGs, about which more information will be given later.

EFAs are a vital part of the structure of all cells, not least of which are those of the skin, 1 square inch (6 square centimetres) of which contains almost 20,000,000. For smooth, supple, non-greasy skin and healthy hair and nails, you need an adequate supply of EFAs.

EFAs also help strengthen the membranes of cells and tiny blood vessels called capillaries, and prevent an increase in skin permeability (see Chapter 9) and consequent moisture loss. In addition, they are required for the control of tissue inflammation. *Other EFA roles.* EFAs play a part in cholesterol metabolism and in blood clotting. They help provide energy, maintain body temperature, insulate nerves, cushion and protect tissues and build resistance to disease.

EFA deficiency
In animal experiments, EFA deficiency produced poor growth and reproductive capacity, lowered energy levels, decreased resistance to certain stresses and various skin inflammations. LA deficiency has led to a breakdown in skin integrity, resulting in certain eczematous conditions.

Other symptoms of EFA deficiency include heart and blood

circulation abnormalities, faulty healing of wounds, abnormal brain development, dried-up tear ducts and salivary glands, impaired resistance to infections and improper formation of collagen, the cement-like material that holds body cells together.

Some experts believe that certain EFA deficiency symptoms may be due to a related prostaglandin (PG) deficiency, since EFAs are precursors of prostaglandins.

In growing animals, a total deprivation of EFAs leads to some serious abnormalities:

— Hair falls out and the skin develops a type of eczema. The sebaceous glands hypertrophy (thicken excessively).

— All body membranes become exceptionally permeable (allowing fluids to pass through), particularly the skin, which loses its ability to prevent water loss. Simultaneously, there is increased thirst, yet despite increased fluid intake, the urine is concentrated.

— The exocrine glands (see Chapter 1), salivary and lacrimal (tear) glands atrophy, or waste away.

— The body's natural defence (immune) system becomes defective, making it more vulnerable to infections.

— Connective tissue formation is impaired and normal healing processes are either delayed or do not occur.

In the 1950s, when a great deal of research was being done on artificial milk preparations for infants, the EFA levels in some formulations were far too low. The Food and Agriculture Organization (FAO) and the World Health Organization (WHO) suggested that a minimum of three per cent of total calories be obtained from EFAs for adults and five per cent for children and pregnant and breast-feeding women.

Infants fed formulae not in keeping with these suggestions developed certain problems: their skin became dry and scaly and eczema-like rashes appeared. The youngsters became very irritable and had much larger appetites than infants of similar age whose feeds contained an adequate supply of EFAs. All the symptoms cleared up, however, when EFAs were added to the deficient formulae.

In the 1970s, when fluids were being developed for long-term intravenous feeding, the American Food and Drug Administration prohibited EFAs from being added to them. The result: a series of reports of acute EFA deficiency in adults who developed skin rashes resembling psoriasis, a type of eczema.

Doctors and authoritative national and international committees have repeatedly encouraged the intake of 10–15 per cent of total calories in the form of EFAs. This contrasts sharply with the 1 per cent total calorie intake which is adequate for young animals to grow and develop normally.

The EFAs are the only nutrients that the medical profession has consistently advised patients to take in large (mega) doses, especially those suffering from heart and blood vessel abnormalities, diabetes, menstrual cycle problems and multiple sclerosis. When doctors urge their clients to increase their polyunsaturate intake, they are referring to EFAs, particularly to linoleic acid (LA).

EFAs and PUFAs
The beneficial effects of polyunsaturated fatty acids (PUFAs) seem to be due to their EFA content. All EFAs are PUFAs, but not all PUFAs are EFAs and the non-EFA PUFAs should be considered saturated in terms of health risks.

Food sources of EFAs
Generally, the best food sources of EFAs are the oils of certain seeds and nuts, the richest being flax seed oil, according to Udo Erasmus.

Specific EFA sources are as follows:

— LA is obtained from certain seed oils, including safflower, sunflower, sesame, corn, soyabean and evening primrose — all rich sources of this EFA. Palm and coconut oil have virtually none; peanut oil has a moderate amount and olive oil only a little.

— Alpha-linolenic acid, which is the same as LNA, is found in green leafy vegetables, in soy oil in small amounts, and in large amounts in linseed oil which Udo Erasmus refers to as the North American version of flax seed oil — the richest source of this EFA.

— Gamma-linolenic acid (GLA). The only truly dependable sources of this very important EFA are human milk and *Efamol* evening primrose oil, and for non-breastfeeding individuals the choice seems clear.

— Dihomo-gamma-linolenic acid (DGLA) is found in small amounts in human milk and in some organ meats, such as kidneys.

— Arachidonic acid (from French 'arachides' meaning 'peanuts') is found in peanuts, of course, and in meats, dairy products, some seaweeds, shrimps and prawns.

More than meets the eye

There seems no shortage of food sources of EFAs and few human diets are such that less than one per cent of the calories consists of LA. It's therefore tempting to conclude that widespread EFA deficiency is a myth. This is faulty reasoning, however, because there's more to this EFA connection than meets the eye.

The only form of LA that can convert into a biologically usable state is what chemists call the 'cis' form. In this case it would be 'cis-linoleic acid', found in unrefined vegetable oils, and of course in evening primrose oil. Once the unadulterated oil has been hydrogenated or otherwise processed, however, the biologically active 'cis' form is turned into the biologically inactive 'trans' form, becoming a 'trans fatty acid'.

'It is unfortunate,' writes a leading researcher and expert on the subject, 'that many doctors are unaware of the existence of trans fatty acids.' One example of this lack of awareness is the advice given to patients to use margarine instead of butter.

'If margarines are recommended,' the researcher adds, 'it is important to insist that they contain PUFAs in which the cis bonds remain intact . . .' (see Bibliography: Horrobin).

Processed vegetable oils are the major source of trans fatty acids in the diet. These products have better keeping properties, or longer shelf life if you wish, than their unprocessed counterparts. Most margarines and vegetable cooking fats contain 20–50 per cent trans PUFAs. Trans PUFAs are also now found in substantial amounts in all processed edibles, including baked goods, sweets and fried foods — commodities frequently consumed by today's busy persons who are usually in a hurry.

Whenever estimates of total human intake of LA have been made, the useful 'cis' and the useless 'trans' forms have been considered together as is of equal value. Consequently, *actual* cis-linoleic acid content has been greatly overestimated.

Herein, then, lies the fallacy that because you step up your polyunsaturate intake by consuming, say, margarine in place of butter, you are proportionately augmenting your supply of cis-linoleic acid.

Trans fatty acids also interfere with an enzyme called delta-6-desaturase (D6D). They also intensify the need for EFAs, probably because of enzyme inhibition. Moreover, they tend to raise the cholesterol level in the blood and so ultimately impair tissue nutrition.

The delta-6-desaturase enzyme

An enzyme, according to the best definition I've yet seen, is 'a biochemical processing device'. You may also consider an enzyme as a catalyst, or helper, which assists in the conversion of one biochemical substance to another.

The enzyme called delta-6-desaturase, or D6D, which you will meet again when the EFA metabolic pathway is described, is vital for the conversion of cis-linoleic acid to gamma-linolenic acid, or GLA. If anything is wrong with D6D, the body may be unable to make normal use of the LA obtained in the diet.

Researchers have discovered that:

— saturated fats inhibit the activity of D6D;

— trans fatty acids, formed by the processing of vegetable oils, also inhibit it;

— in diabetic animals, the activity of this enzyme is low;

— alcohol inhibits it;

— ageing contributes to loss of the enzyme activity;

— adrenalin, a hormone intimately involved in stress inhibits D6D;

— starvation inhibits the enzyme, but cutting down on calories may actually increase its activity three-fold;

— a very low protein intake inhibits D6D, but a very high protein intake activates it;

— viruses with the potential to cause cancer and some forms of radiation inhibit the enzyme.

It is thus apparent that many agents that adversely affect good health (e.g. alcohol, some forms of dieting, diabetes, 'stress hormones') also influence the D6D enzyme. These factors seem to reduce the availability of EFAs to the body through their effects on the enzyme, a fact that has seemingly escaped many researchers.

Before describing the EFA metabolic pathway, mentioned earlier, it seems opportune to discuss prostaglandins, a word you'll be meeting again and again.

The PG factor

Prostaglandins (PGs), so called because they were first reported as a component of secretions of the prostate gland, are in fact made by practically every tissue in the body. They are sometimes referred to as local hormones.

These fatty acid molecules are an integral part of the membrane surrounding each cell, and local disturbances near a cell can result in their release from the membrane. Once released, they are then converted into their active prostaglandin (PG) forms which, though shortlived, profoundly affect various body functions. Much of their effect depends not only on their amount, but also on their type and ratios. Often, it is the balance and combination of PGs that determine the efficient functioning of a particular organ.

Seven types of PGs have so far been identified and, like vitamins, they have been given letter names: E, F, A, B, C and D.

Some PGs generate pain, and many anti-prostaglandin medications are now marketed to inhibit this distressing PG function.

But there are good PGs as well, and prostaglandin E1, or PGE1, is one of them. In fact, PGE1 may be considered a 'superprostaglandin'.

PGE1

Listed below are some of the apparent actions of PGE1:

— it dilates, or gives greater diameter, to blood vessels, thus improving blood flow to the skin, scalp and other parts of the body which depend on it for nourishment;

— it helps prevent cholesterol build-up, so that blood vessels remain sufficiently patent (wide open) to permit unrestricted blood flow;

— it counteracts inflammations;

— it discourages abnormal cell proliferation, that is, a too-rapid increase;

— it regulates the immune system, which is the body's natural defence against infections and other forms of disease.

The EFA Metabolic Pathway

Earlier, it was pointed out that although there's no shortage of food sources of the EFA, linoleic acid (LA), this nutrient has to be in the 'cis' form before it can successfully pass through the series of chemical reactions necessary for its effective utilization by the body.

As a nutrient, LA has no biological activity on its own. Its value lies in the fact that it is the raw material from which active ingredients can be made, the final being PGE1.

Think of the series of chemical reactions from cis-linoleic acid to PGE1 as a sort of race. Cis-linoleic acid, the starter substance, represents the starting line, PGE1 is the finishing line and the entire 'race' consists of three stages (Figure 3).

The first stage of this imaginary race consists of the conversion of cis-linoleic acid to a substance called gamma-linolenic acid (GLA). No matter how much LA there is in the diet, it is useless if it cannot be converted into GLA, and there are many agents — obstacles if you like — that can prevent this conversion. These are sometimes referred to as 'blocking agents', and their favourite site is stage one of the metabolic 'track', that is, between LA and GLA (see Figure 3).

Blocking agents

Blocking agents preventing the conversion of cis-linoleic acid to GLA include:

— defective or deficient D6D, described earlier in this chapter;

Figure 3: EFA Metabolic Pathway

CIS-LINOLEIC ACID

↓

enzyme delta-6-desaturase needed

↓

helped by
biotin, magnesium, vitamin B_6, zinc

blocked by
ageing, alcohol (moderate to high
intake), diabetes, high-cholesterol
foods, magnesium, pyridoxine and
zinc deficiencies, saturated fats,
trans fatty acids, virus infections
and cancer

↓

GAMMA-LINOLENIC ACID (GLA)
(from Evening Primrose Oil)

helped by
vitamin B_6

↓

DIHOMO-GAMMALINOLENIC ACID (DGLA)

helped by
vitamin B_3, vitamin C, zinc

↓

PROSTAGLANDIN E1

— high-cholesterol foods;

— foods abundant in trans fatty acids, for example, oils subjected to high heat, deodorized, hydrogenated or otherwise artificially processed; pastries, sweets and French fries;

— moderate to high alcohol intake;

— deficiencies of magnesium, pyridoxine (vitamin B_6) and zinc;

— diabetes;

— ageing;

— virus infections, radiation and cancer.

By now you will have come to appreciate more fully why, although you may be eating adequately foods providing an ample supply of EFAs, these nutrients may not in fact be available to the tissues. This should come as no surprise considering the proliferation of highly processed foods now being habitually consumed by millions of busy persons in affluent countries such as ours.

Co-factors

On the metabolic pathway from cis-linoleic acid to PGE1, certain enzymes, vitamins and minerals are needed to facilitate passage from one stage to the next. Scientists refer to these as 'co-factors', and they may be thought of as friendly helpers along the way.

Notable among these are the enzyme D6D, the B-complex vitamins particularly biotin, vitamin B_3 (niacin) and vitamin B_6 (pyridoxine), as well as vitamin C, magnesium and zinc. These nutrients are dealt with in detail in the next chapter in connection with the nourishment of the hair, skin and nails. A deficiency of any of them could adversely affect satisfactory EFA metabolism.

Gamma-linolenic acid

Whereas other EFAs need to progress through all the stages of the metabolic pathway to PGE1, gamma-linolenic acid (GLA) does not. It starts the metabolic 'race' not at the starting line, but rather at the beginning of the second stage. This puts it at an advantage since it does not encounter the blocking agents frequently present in stage one.

It so happens that GLA is the active ingredient of an oil that has been in existence for a very long time, and which is once again enjoying well deserved recognition. It is the seed oil of the evening primrose flower, and I have devoted all of Chapter 4 to it.

A particularly dependable form of evening primrose oil, used internationally in over 200 clinical trials to date, is *Efamol*. Its mineral/vitamin companion, *Efavite*, contains four of the co-factors needed for the successful conversion of cis-linoleic acid to PGE1.

So, with a reliable source of GLA available, the metabolic race can continue unhindered through stages two and three to the PGE1 'finish line', provided that the necessary co-factors are supplied (see Figure 3).

3. An ABC of Skin Nutrition

No isolated nutrient can bear the body's entire nutritional load. All nutrients work together, and to single out one of them and expect it to work miracles is, according to the late Adelle Davis, like playing chess with nothing but a bishop.

Having stated this, I shall, in this chapter, focus the spotlight on several nutrients that are of particular significance to the health and attractiveness of the skin, and to the hair and nails which are modified forms of skin.

Vitamins

Vitamin A

Vitamin A, sometimes called the 'skin vitamin', is a fat-soluble vitamin needed for young-looking skin and healthy hair and nails.

When this nutrient is undersupplied, cells in the lower layers of skin die and slough off. They plug oil sacs and pores and so prevent oil from reaching the skin surface. The skin may then become dry, rough and itchy. Roughness is first noticeable on the elbows and knees. Whiteheads, blackheads and pimples may appear, and the skin may become vulnerable to infections such as boils.

These conditions can usually be corrected, however, by increasing vitamin A intake, provided other essential nutrients are amply supplied in the diet. Tests have demonstrated that vitamin A can indeed discourage premature ageing of skin and other tissues by preventing the breakdown of cell membranes.

Vitamin A has been shown to enhance the conversion of GLA to PGE1, substances that play a major role in normal skin function, and which are known to decrease with age (see Chapter 2).

Vitamin A is also well documented as playing an important part in the differentiation of epithelial cells during skin growth. This means that it is needed to help cells develop in form or character according to their specific function, which may differ from that of surrounding cells.

Research has now established that cell oxygenation — whereby cells are supplied with oxygen — is enhanced by vitamin A combined with vitamin E. Another important vitamin A function is to increase the permeability of the tiny blood vessels (capillaries) that carry oxygen and other health- and life-supporting nutrients to every single cell. (Capillary permeability exists when the capillary wall allows blood to pass readily into cells or tissue spaces, or vice versa.) The more permeable the capillary walls, the better the oxygen supply delivered to the cells and the more 'youthful' the tissues they form. Efficient cell oxygenation is one of the secrets of young-looking skin.

Recently, a vitamin A derivative in cream form has been widely publicized as a marvelous antidote to wrinkles. It is called tretinoin (Retin-A, or vitamin A acid), and many dermatologists find that it is their most frequently prescribed drug. It was, originally, a topical treatment for acne, and a very effective one. Prescribing topical tretinoin as an anti-wrinkle cream is now considered 'accepted medical practice'. Indeed, scientific evidence indicates that it does reverse photodamage to the skin.

People who use this product should be aware that it does make the stratum corneum thinner. The skin is therefore more sensitive to sunlight than usual. The use of a sunscreen and other protection are consequently very important. Moreover, topical tretinoin used to counteract wrinkles must be a life-long treatment in order to maintain the benefits gained.

Vitamin A deficiency can result in dry, dull hair and an accumulation of dandruff. It causes the scalp to thicken so that it traps oil and perspiration beneath the surface. A vitamin A-deficient diet may, in addition, cause ridges to appear on the nails, which may also peel, split, break off, fail to grow or become exceedingly thin.

Vitamin A is obtained, ready made, from foods of animal origin and from plant sources in the form of carotene which is converted into the vitamin in the body.

Good vegetable sources of this nutrient include broccoli, carrots, dandelion leaves and other dark green leafy vegetables such as turnip greens, as well as endive, parsley, sweet potatoes, tomatoes, winter squash and the 'pot liquor' or cooking liquid, from these vegetables which is unfortunately often discarded. Fresh fruits highest in vitamin A are apricots, cantaloupe melons, cherries, mangoes, mulberries, nectarines, papayas and peaches. Other vitamin A sources are dairy products, eggs, fish and fish liver oils.

Vitamin A, like all other vitamins and essential fatty acids, absorbs well through the skin.

Caution: As with other fat-soluble vitamins, excessive vitamin A in the diet can produce undesirable side effects. Among these are dry skin and inflammation of hair follicles, with consequent hair loss. These conditions are reversible, though, once consumption of the vitamin is reduced to normal.

The B vitamins

The B vitamins are a complex of over a dozen water-soluble vitamins that help to build and repair the body's cells and produce resilient skin. They are sometimes called the 'nerve vitamins' and are of particular value in helping counteract the harmful effects of high stress levels.

It seems appropriate at this point to mention that during the first few weeks of our pre-natal development, what would later become our hair, skin, nails and pituitary and adrenal glands were all part of the *ectoderm*. This is the name given to the outer layer of cells in an embryo, which is what we were between the second and eighth weeks of our life before birth. Knowing this may help you appreciate why some skin disorders occur when we suffer from nervous conditions such as anxiety and depression.

Vitamin B$_2$

Vitamin B$_2$ (riboflavin), which is especially important to skin tissue, helps in the transportation of oxygen and is vital to carbohydrate metabolism. When riboflavin is deficient in the diet, the lips may become lined, as when puckered for whistling, the wrinkles being most noticeable when the face is relaxed.

In volunteers who stayed on diets lacking this vitamin, the skin of the forehead, nose and chin became oily and tiny fatty deposits like whiteheads accumulated under the skin. Fissures appeared at the corners of the mouth and eyelids, and the eyelashes stuck together with an oily secretion, especially when the subjects awoke in the morning. Cracks and oily scabs formed at the base of the nose. Oily hair is another sign of a riboflavin-deficient diet. Nerve function is impaired as well, and the body becomes more vulnerable to infection.

Foods rich in riboflavin include almonds, Brewer's yeast, broccoli, dark green leafy vegetables, eggs, legumes (dried peas, beans and lentils), Lima beans, milk and milk products, sunflower seeds, wheatgerm and wild rice.

Vitamin B$_3$

Vitamin B$_3$ (niacin) helps to maintain healthy blood circulation, by means of which the hair, skin and nails receive their nourishment. Niacin is also important for a sound nervous system, and we know that the skin is abundantly supplied with nerve endings (see Chapter 1).

Niacin is a co-factor in the metabolism of EFAs, helping to convert DGLA to PGE1 (see Chapter 2).

A niacin-deficient diet has been linked with certain forms of dermatitis (skin inflammation). In some persons suffering even mild niacin deficiency, a skin condition resembling sunburn appears. Later, the skin may darken and become dry and scaly.

Good food sources of niacin are artichokes, asparagus, Brewer's yeast, fish, green leafy vegetables, legumes, nuts, potatoes, seafood, seeds, whole grains and whole grain products.

Vitamin B₅

Vitamin B₅ (pantothenic acid or calcium pantothenate) is regarded as an anti-dermatitis factor, important for healthy skin. Every body cell needs it, and neither carbohydrates (sugars and starches) nor fats can be changed into energy without it.

This nutrient is also important for the normal functioning of the adrenal glands, located above the kidneys. The secretions of the adrenals play a very important role in stress, which in turn affects the health and appearance of the skin, hair and nails. Indeed, pantothenic acid has been called the 'anti-stress vitamin'.

When simultaneous deficiencies of pantothenic acid and vitamin B₆ were produced in volunteers, pain similar to that from sunburn was experienced, and eczema appeared on the face, arms, scrotum and other parts of the body. It took three weeks for the symptoms to respond to treatment with the appropriate vitamin supplements.

Other volunteers in whom pantothenic acid deficiencies were induced became more vulnerable to infection and adrenal gland exhaustion than they would normally have been.

In animals lacking this nutrient, hair turns grey and hair bulbs and follicles atrophy (waste away).

Good food sources of pantothenic acid include avocados, Brewer's yeast, broccoli, cabbage, cashew nuts, cauliflower, corn, egg yolk, Filbert nuts, green vegetables, milk, molasses, mushrooms, peanuts, pecan nuts, potatoes, salmon, sunflower seeds, trout, unrefined vegetable oils and whole grains.

Vitamin B₆

Vitamin B₆ (pyridoxine) plays a major role in the body's utilization of carbohydrates and fats, in the normal functioning of skin and nerves and in the production of hormones.

Pyridoxine is necessary for the production of antibodies which protect against infection, and also aids in the formation of red blood cells. It activates many enzyme systems and plays an important part in protein metabolism. Popular high protein diets, for instance, increase the body's need for this nutrient.

In fat (lipid) metabolism, pyridoxine plays a vital role, particularly in connection with the EFAs. It is a co-factor which facilitates the conversion of LA to GLA and GLA to DGLA (see Chapter 2). It is essential for the utilization of LA.

Pyridoxine is also required for proper carbohydrate metabolism and to regulate the crucial balance between the minerals sodium (salt) and potassium. It is also essential for the maintenance of normal magnesium levels in the blood and tissues, and neither of these nutrients can work without the other.

A pyridoxine deficiency produces sore, cracked lips, excessively oily skin and dandruff. In men whose diets were deficient of this nutrient, dry, scaly skin resulted, and a rash accompanied by itching appeared on the scrotum. Dandruff was also abundant.

The symptoms took two weeks to clear up with vitamin B_6 and magnesium supplementation (the latter decreases the body's need for the former).

Good pyridoxine sources include avocados, bananas, Brewer's yeast, buckwheat flour, carrots, eggs, Filbert nuts, fresh fish, milk, prunes, raisins, rice (brown), sunflower seeds, tomatoes, wheatgerm, whole grains and whole grain products.

Vitamin B_9

Vitamin B_9 (folic acid) is vital for the formation of healthy red blood cells and for keeping the body's natural defence (immune) system in good working order. It also plays a part in the utilization of fats.

A folic acid deficiency may result in anaemia ('iron-poor blood') and consequently, impaired nutrient to the body's cells. Hair, including the eyebrows and eyelashes, may fall out.

Folic acid may also play a part in the maintenance and restoration of normal hair colour.

When this nutrient is undersupplied in the diet, the skin may become blemished, and a greyish-brown pigmentation may result. This is sometimes seen in pregnancy and is called 'pregnancy cap'. It does respond, however, to supplementation with the vitamin.

Frequent hangnails are yet another sign that folic acid, together with vitamin C and protein, is deficient.

Brewer's yeast, green leafy vegetables, green onions, tempeh (a sort of cheese made from fermented soya beans), wheatgerm and whole grain products are among the richest sources of folic acid.

Biotin

Biotin, sometimes called vitamin H, is a nutrient associated with the B-complex group of vitamins. It stimulates the growth of body cells and is related to hair growth.

In experimental animals, a biotin deficiency produced inflamed skin, eczema, grey hair and hair loss almost to the point of baldness.

Biotin is a co-factor in EFA metabolism. It helps convert LA to GLA (see Chapter 2).

The chief food sources of this nutrient are Brewer's yeast, desiccated liver, eggs, fish, legumes, milk, nuts, wheatgerm and whole grains.

Inositol

Inositol, another B-complex member, occurs naturally in the brain and muscles. With the exception of niacin, there is more inositol in the body than any other vitamin.

In laboratory animals, a diet deficient in inositol produced baldness. In humans, treatment with inositol, together with other B vitamins, has arrested or reversed hair loss. Inositol deficiency has also produced eczema.

Brewer's yeast is an excellent source of inositol. Barley, blackstrap molasses, cantaloupe melons, grapefruit, legumes, nuts, oats, oranges, seeds, wheatgerm, whole grains and whole grain products are all good sources.

PABA

PABA (para amino benzoic acid) was first publicized as an anti-grey-hair vitamin. Scientists have been able to produce grey hair in dark-haired animals by withholding PABA from their diet. When the animals were fed the missing PABA, normal hair colour returned.

One researcher was able to achieve similar results in humans.

Dr Benjamin Sieve studied the hair of persons given 200 milligrams of PABA after each meal. In 70 per cent of the cases, some hair was restored to its natural colour.

Persons who become easily sunburned were able to tolerate considerable more sunshine after supplementation with PABA.

In animals lacking this vitamin, dermatitis has resulted. In humans, the nutrient has been used successfully, again and again, to clear up a wide variety of eczemas.

Like other B-complex vitamins, PABA is amply supplied by Brewer's yeast, eggs, molasses and whole grains.

About Brewer's yeast. You will have noted that Brewer's yeast repeatedly occurs as a food source of the B vitamins and for good reasons.

Dr Paavo Airola (see Bibliography) recommends true Brewer's yeast — rather than torula or nutritional yeasts — as the best source of the B vitamins as well as various trace minerals such as selenium and zinc, and high quality protein. He also points out that Brewer's yeast is possibly the best source of the *nucleic acids*, substances directly involved in cell rejuvenation to help keep us youthful.

To avoid problems with gas, it's best to mix one tablespoon (15 ml) of Brewer's yeast powder in half a glass of freshly made pineapple, grapefruit or other acid juice, and take it two or three times daily one hour before meals.

Brewer's yeast should always be taken on an empty stomach, when there is a rich supply of the stomach's hydrochloric acid to digest it properly.

Because Brewer's yeast is high in phosphorus and relatively low in calcium, it's wise to take a calcium supplement with it to achieve a better mineral balance and improve utilization of the nutrients.

Vitamin C

Vitamin C, or ascorbic acid, is also known as the 'anti-scorbutic', or 'anti-scurvy', vitamin. It is water soluble and needed for healthy tissues, to promote healing and to reinforce the body's resistance to disease.

Vitamin C is essential for the formation and maintenance of the strong cement-like material known as *collagen* (see Chapter 1). Collagen holds together all the cells in your body, and the amount required uses about one-third of all the body's protein.

Collagen serves much the same purpose as cement does in a brick building, except that the 'concrete' in a healthy body is in the form of a gristle-like gelatin called connective tissue. This tissue gives strength and elasticity to all the structures it supports. When vitamin C is undersupplied in the diet, this foundation weakens and the skin begins to sag.

Hangnails occur frequently when the diet is deficient in this very important nutrient.

Research has shown that a vitamin C deficiency leads to collagen deterioration. When this occurs, wrinkles, flabbiness, skin discoloration and other signs of ageing appear. Adequate vitamin C intake will keep collagen healthy and preserve the tensile strength of all the body's tissues. This will, among other benefits, contribute to skin that's firm and attractive. Vitamin C also plays a part in the blood circulation and the utilization of oxygen.

Studies have shown that many manifestations of old age — for example, dry skin, wrinkles and loss of tissue elasticity — are actually signs of scurvy, which is due to a vitamin C deficiency. Certainly, observed nutritionist Adelle Davis, persons wishing to retain youthfulness should see that their vitamin C intake is ample.

Interestingly, some North American coastal Indian tribes used the evening primrose plant as an anti-scorbutic. Haida women, in particular, considered it a valuable beauty aid.

Vitamin C is a co-factor in EFA metabolism. It helps convert DGLA to PGE1 (see Chapter 2). Since our bodies cannot synthesize this vitamin, we need to obtain it every day from the diet or from supplements. The best vegetable sources of vitamin C are cabbage, dandelion leaves, green and red peppers, kohlrabi, mustard and cress, turnip tops; but all fresh vegetables, particularly if eaten raw, will contribute to your vitamin C intake.

The best fruit sources of vitamin C are apricots, blackberries, cantaloupe melons, cherries, elderberries, gooseberries, grape-fruit, guavas, honeydew melons, kumquats, lemons, limes, oranges, papayas, rosehips and strawberries.

About rosehips. In his book entitled *Everywoman's Book. Dr. Airola's Guide to Holistic Health* (see Bibliography), the doctor has written about the gorgeous complexion of the Swedish people. He has attributed this, in large part, to their liberal use of rosehips.

Rosehips are the berries of the wild rose bush. The Swedes apparently gather these in the late fall and use them to make desserts, jellies, soups and teas. They also buy them in super-markets and health food stores where they are readily available.

Rosehips, writes Dr Airola, are perhaps the richest known source of vitamin C (acerola, or Caribbean cherries, excepted), containing between twenty and forty times as much vitamin C as oranges. They are also exceedingly rich in the *bioflavonoids*, substances that enhance the action of vitamin C, and which are also known as vitamin P.

Vitamin D

Vitamin D facilitates the absorption and utilization of calcium. Until recently, it was believed that adults had adequate reserves of this vitamin in their tissues, and that sunshine was the best source.

Our most reliable source of this vitamin, however, is vitamin D-enriched milk. Butter, eggs and fish liver oils contain small amounts. Plant foods contain no vitamin D.

Vitamin E

The major function of this fat-soluble vitamin seems to be to prevent unsaturated fatty acids and other fat-like substances from being destroyed by oxygen. These substances include vitamin A, carotene, EFAs and various hormones.

Vitamin E is also necessary for the formation of the nucleus of every cell in the body, and when you consider that in a mere square inch (6 square centimetres) of skin there are almost 20,000,000 cells, you will readily understand how crucial this nutrient is to the health of the skin, our largest organ.

Vitamin E is an anti-oxidant. It averts certain types of oxygen damage from key body constituents, notably fats. When vitamin E is deficient, EFAs combine with oxygen and break down. And since EFAs are now known to form not only part of the internal structure and wall of all cells but also the connective tissue between them, it is not difficult to appreciate the importance of vitamin E in this respect.

World renowned expert on stress, Dr Hans Selye, has referred to vitamin E as one of our basic anti-stress vitamins. It improves blood circulation and prevents harmful oxidation of fats by increasing the oxygen supply to cells and tissues. In animal experiments, Dr Selye was able to bring on signs and symptoms of old age by withholding vitamin E from the test animals. Through the use of vitamin E, he was able to prolong life and youthfulness in other animals.

Vitamin E reduces the production of *leukotrienes*, potentially harmful products of EFA chemistry.

In addition, vitamin E plays an important role in the transport, absorption and storage of vitamin A in the body. In animal experiments, vitamin A absorption was severely impaired when the diet was deficient in vitamin E. When oral vitamin E supplements were given, the animals' ability to use vitamin A increased six-fold.

Vitamin E has been used successfully in the treatment of scar tissue. In London, Canada, the scars of burn victims healed without contraction, itching and intense pain after treatment with the vitamin. In some cases, even old, unsightly scars disappeared.

Although healthy skin is amazingly elastic, some persons who have lost a great deal of weight, and many women who have borne children, develop stretch marks. Vitamin E has proven of value in helping these unattractive marks to fade. In some cases of premature ageing, large amounts of vitamin E have helped prevent wrinkle formation.

The body's vitamin E requirements increase when EFA intake is high and when iron supplements are being used. A few words of caution about iron, however: if you frequently use enriched white bread and cereals, be aware that these usually contain an inorganic form of iron which combines with vitamin E and destroys it. Also, you should *not* take mineral supplements containing inorganic iron, *unless* you take the vitamin E and the mineral supplement eight hours apart. Preferable forms of iron are ferrous gluconate, ferrous fumarate, peptonized iron and iron lactate, since these are organic.

Vitamin E has been described as a protector against disturbing environmental influences, such as sunlight. Scientific evidence has shown that taking 400 International Units (IU) daily of d-alpha tocopheryl acetate or d-alpha tocopheryl acid succinate — *not* the 'dl' form, which is far less active — and the trace mineral selenium (100 micrograms daily) can decrease skin damage by the sun. In addition, these two substances have been proven to decrease the incidence of various cancers, including skin cancer. Taking four or five vitamin E tablets as soon as possible after severe sunburn will also help decrease inflammation.

X-ray and other radiation treatments are known to destroy not only vitamin E, but also vitamins A, C, several B vitamins and the EFAs. The destruction of vitamin E and the EFAs can, however, be largely prevented if ample supplies of vitamin E are provided.

Good vitamin E sources include almonds and other nuts, broccoli, eggs, fruits, green leafy vegetables, legumes, seeds, unrefined vegetable oils, wheatgerm and whole grains. (When oils are refined or hydrogenated, vitamin E is completely lost.)

Evening primrose oil is a substantial source of vitamin E. A further 13.6 International Units (IU) have been added to each *Efamol* evening primrose oil capsule to ensure that intake of this very important nutrient is indeed ample.

Minerals

Minerals are essential constituents of all cells and form the greater portion of the hard parts of the body such as the nails. They are important catalysts (helpers) in biological reactions and transmitters of nerve impulses.

The processing of foods substantially alters their mineral

content, raising the phosphorus level in many cases and lowering that of several other essential minerals such as magnesium and zinc. Flour is a good example: 75 per cent of the iron, magnesium, potassium and zinc are lost in its refining.

Calcium

Calcium is needed for the proper functioning of nervous tissue, for good muscle tone and for normal blood clotting. It is considered an anti-stress mineral and is required as well for a sound chemical balance in the body.

It is common knowledge that calcium is needed for healthy bones and teeth. Not so well known, though, is the fact that calcium is closely linked to the metabolism (the production of the energy by which we live and move) of EFAs which are vital to the health of hair, skin and nails.

Emotional stress and prolonged bedrest increase our calcium requirements, as do high protein and high fat diets. Calcium also plays a part in wound healing. The scar tissue that forms when wounds and injuries heal is a connective tissue made of collagen, which depends on both vitamin C and calcium for strength. Calcium has also been used successfully to relieve the itching of a skin eruption called hives.

Vitamin D supplies must be adequate for calcium to be properly absorbed. Vitamin C and milk sugar (lactose) enhance calcium absorption. Blackstrap molasses, carob flour (the ground seed pods of a Mediterranean tree which resembles cocoa or chocolate), citrus fruits, dried figs, green vegetables, milk and milk products and sesame seeds are among the best calcium sources. Good calcium supplements are also available in health food stores.

Copper

Copper is an essential trace mineral which plays an important role in many enzyme systems. It is vital for the production of RNA (ribonucleic acid), which is part of the nucleus of every cell. It helps in the development and function of nerve, brain and connective tissue, and it is needed in small amounts to help synthesize haemoglobin, the colouring matter of red blood cells.

Copper also plays a part in pigment formation. Black animals lacking copper become grey and in humans, greying has been linked to anaemia associated with a copper deficiency.

According to one dermatologist, copper is a component of an enzyme that gives hair its structure. Without copper in the diet, abnormalities of the hair shaft can occur, causing the hair to lose its tensile quality.

Copper deficiency decreases the absorption of iron, shortens the life span of red blood cells and so contributes to anaemia. In animals, a lack of copper results in hair loss, skin rash and degeneration of the myelin sheath (the fatty covering of nerve fibres).

According to Adelle Davis, author of *Let's Eat Right to Keep Fit* (see Bibliography), copper is richest in the least popular meats, namely liver, kidneys and brain. Oysters and nuts are also very good sources. Small amounts are found in green leafy vegetables grown on fertile soils, lentils and whole grain breads and cereals.

Iron

Iron is a vital component of haemoglobin, the red colouring matter of blood, by means of which oxygen is transported to all body cells. Iron is also an important part of numerous enzyme systems and plays a role in the nutrition of epithelial tissues.

An iron deficiency results in anaemia, signs and symptoms of which include pallor of the skin, fingernail beds and mucous membranes. Other manifestations of an undersupply of iron are nails that are brittle and show longitudinal ridging.

According to Adelle Davis, the greatest single cause of iron-deficiency anaemia is the refining of breads, cereals and sugar. She further points out that, although much has been said about the iron in so-called enriched flour, this food item is not a rich source of iron compared, for example, with Brewer's yeast and wheatgerm.

Because only a fraction of the iron present in food is absorbed, it is necessary to provide between 15 and 30 mg (milligrams) in the diet to ensure that 1 to 4 mg (normal range of adult requirements) will be absorbed.

The best vegetable sources of iron include green leafy vegetables, legumes and seaweed. Fruits richest in iron include dried fruit, Sharon fruit (persimmon) and watermelon. Other dietary sources are blackstrap molasses, Brewer's yeast, cereals (unrefined), egg yolk, ocean perch, sardines, shellfish and whole grains.

In order for iron to be satisfactorily absorbed, three trace minerals must be present in the diet. These are cobalt, found in crab, oysters and sardines; copper (see previous section on copper), and manganese, supplied by green leafy vegetables, nuts, unrefined grains grown on healthy soils, wheat bran and wheatgerm.

Magnesium

Magnesium is a mineral needed by every cell in the body. It is essential for the synthesis of protein and for the utilization of fats, the B vitamins, vitamin E and several minerals. It is also an important catalyst in many enzyme reactions. Most of these enzymes also contain vitamin B_6, which is not well absorbed unless magnesium is generously supplied in the diet. In fact, these two nutrients are so interdependent that neither can function effectively without the other.

Magnesium, as mentioned earlier, decreases the body's need for vitamin B_6. It has been used successfully, in conjunction with the vitamin, to clear up certain troublesome skin problems (see section on vitamin B_6).

The best natural sources of magnesium are alfalfa sprouts, almonds and other nuts eaten fresh from the shell, beetroot tops, blackstrap molasses, brown rice, celery, chard, dried fruits, grapefruit, green leafy vegetables, especially kale, grown on mineral-rich soils, oranges, potatoes, peas, sesame seeds, shellfish, soyabeans, sunflower seeds, wheat bran, wheatgerm and whole grains.

The milling of grains has substantially affected our magnesium intake. White flour, for example, has only about 22 per cent of the magnesium found in wholewheat flour. The bran and germ of wheat — valuable sources of this nutrient — are removed during milling.

Selenium

This trace mineral is needed to maintain satisfactory blood circulation and to reinforce the body's natural defence against disease (immune system). Selenium works, along with vitamins C and E, to help keep the body free of potentially harmful substances. A selenium deficiency has been linked to premature ageing and high blood-pressure.

Good sources of this nutrient are asparagus, Brewer's yeast, eggs, garlic, mushrooms, seafood and whole grains.

Silicon

Some skin experts say that this trace mineral gives life to the skin, lustre to the hair and beautiful finishing touches to the whole body. Silicon is also required for healthy connective tissue and normal functioning of the adrenal glands.

Foods made from natural buckwheat are a particularly rich source of this micro-nutrient. Other sources include asparagus, carrots, celery, eggs, green pepper, lentils, lettuce, liver, oats and other whole grains, mushrooms, parsley, pumpkin, strawberries and tomatoes.

Sulphur

Known as 'the beauty mineral', sulphur helps keep the complexion clear and the hair glossy. It also plays a part in cell formation and respiration, and in the synthesis of collagen.

Natural food sources of sulphur include bran, Brussels sprouts, cabbage, horseradish, peppers (all kinds), kale, oats, protein foods and radishes.

Zinc

The trace mineral zinc is intricately involved in tissue nutrition and repair. It is essential for the proper functioning of more than 70 enzyme systems, including the production of hormones and the maintenance of healthy hair, skin and nails.

Zinc deficiencies have resulted in dermatitis (skin inflammation), loss of hair and poor wound healing. Lack of zinc can also interfere with the metabolism of vitamin A, the 'skin vitamin'. Zinc supplements are, in fact, sometimes prescribed for individuals who have undergone surgery.

Zinc, according to Roger J. Williams, author of *Nutrition Against Disease*, (see Bibliography) is an element that has, until recently, received scant attention with regard to its role in human nutrition. In the 1960s, he reports, the Food and Drug Administration of the USA required labels of supplements containing zinc to state that the need for this mineral had not been established. They demanded this despite the fact that, for many years, it was known that zinc is an essential constituent of an indispensable enzyme called *carbonic anhydrase*, and that zinc can be obtained only from the diet or from supplements. (Carbonic anhydrase removes carbon dioxide from tissues.)

Zinc is necessary for the assimilation of the B vitamins, themselves vital to the health of the hair, skin and nails. Zinc is also a co-factor in EFA metabolism. It is needed to convert LA to GLA and DGLA to PGE1 (see Chapter 2).

Zinc deficiencies are far more widespread than recognized and a lack of this nutrient interferes with the formation of the very nucleus of every cell in our body. An undersupply of zinc in humans as well as in animals causes low resistance to infection of all kinds, slow healing and a skin disorder similar to psoriasis (a type of dermatitis).

The November 1979 issue of *Prevention* magazine records a case of a teenage boy who was hospitalized for a severe head injury and had to be tube fed. The youngster developed a facial inflammation and a leg ulcer, both of which cleared up nicely when he was given about 22 mg of zinc daily in the form of supplements.

Zinc has also been used, with some success, in treating a rare, inherited childhood disorder, called AE (acrodermatitis enteropathica). Symptoms of AE include severe skin eruptions and hair loss.

One doctor has reported that treatment with zinc supplements (between 20–40 mg per day) has led to consistent, sustained improvement of this potentially lethal condition.

When physicians in Sweden gave zinc to one of their patients suffering from AE, they noticed that his acne cleared up almost totally. Encouraged, they treated groups of young adults with severe inflammatory acne with zinc, and in about 12 weeks gained remarkable results.

For more details about this important and fascinating micro-nutrient, do read *The Z Factor* by Judy Graham and Dr Michel Odent (see Bibliography).

Proteins

Proteins form the basic structure of every body cell. Your hair, skin and nails are essentially protein. A protein deficiency results in loss of muscle mass and tone, wrinkling of the skin and other signs of ageing.

Fingernails that split or break, fail to grow or are exceedingly thin may be clues to a protein-deficient diet. The rate of nail growth has, in fact, been used to measure protein adequacy.

While sufficient protein in the diet is essential for the health and attractiveness of the hair, skin and nails, an excess increases the demand for other nutrients — vitamin B_6 for example.

The best vegetable protein sources include legumes, nuts and grains such as corn, millet, oats and wheat. To be complete, though, these foods need to be combined at the same meal with complementary proteins containing the amino acids they lack. You will find a wealth of information on protein complementarity in Frances Moore Lappé's *Diet for a Small Planet* (see Bibliography).

Water

Water, though not generally considered a nutrient, is in fact the most important substance we consume. We can survive prolonged fasts, but will almost certainly die after several days without taking in water.

Humans are composed mostly of water. A woman, on average,

is between 55 and 65 per cent water, and a man between 65 and 75 per cent.

Water is the principal constituent of all body fluids (blood, lymph and tissue fluids). It is the medium by which nutrients are carried to all cells and waste products removed through the blood circulatory and lymphatic systems. It is a shock absorber, a temperature regulator and a lubricant.

Deprivation of water or excessive water loss leads to dehydration, with resulting dry skin. When the *stratum corneum* lacks water, skin becomes dry, rough or cracked because this skin layer needs water to maintain its flexibility. (The *stratum corneum* is the skin's outermost layer. It is itself made up of several layers of flattened cells containing *keratin* which prevents water loss from deeper tissues.)

Antagonists

An antagonist is, literally, that which counteracts the action of something else. The following act against the potential good of the vitamins, minerals and other nutrients mentioned in this chapter: contraceptive pills; too much coffee and tea; excessive use of salt, sugar and alcohol; radiation from the sun and from x-rays; high stress levels and lack of regular exercise.

Interestingly, these antagonists also interfere with proper EFA metabolism, as mentioned in Chapter 2, and therefore affect the condition of the hair, skin and nails.

Other vitamin and mineral antagonists include aspirin, which increases the need for vitamin C; rancid foods which destroy vitamin E; some commercial laxatives which cause deficiencies of vitamin C and the B-complex vitamins, and smoking which will be dealt with in detail in Chapter 9.

Conclusion
In no instance, observed Adelle Davis, are nutrient deficiencies more apparent than in abnormalities of the hair, skin and nails. Fortunately, however, the effects of good nutrient are equally obvious.

I hope that the information given in this chapter will help you become more nutrition conscious, and that it will whet your appetite for further related knowledge. For knowledge provides the basis for the intelligent care that will ultimately result in healthier, more attractive hair, skin and nails.

4. EVENING PRIMROSE OIL

When I was a child, I often heard people say that good things come in small packages. Applied to the evening primrose, this saying would undoubtedly be true. For within its tiny seeds, no bigger than those of the mustard plant, there is an oil that has already begun to fulfil promises of being exceptional in the fields of nutrition and medicine.

Botanically known as *Oenothera biennis* (from Greek *oinos*, wine, and *thera*, a hunt), the active principle of the evening primrose plant was thought to counteract the effects of wine, and indeed I recently heard of a case where it prevented a previously inevitable hangover.

Description

The flowers of the evening primrose plant are generally bright yellow and have a delicate fragrance. They usually open between 6 and 7 o'clock in the evening — hence their name. Some plants grow no higher than dandelions. Others shoot up as high as 2 metres, which is about 6 feet.

At special farms in Britain, the plants are being cultivated under controlled conditions to produce varieties that will give the highest yield of oil with the highest GLA levels at the lowest possible cost.

History

For over 500 years, the evening primrose plant was used by natives of North and Central America for a variety of health and beauty purposes. The Haida Indians of British Columbia, Canada, seemed to use it more than any other tribe. They gathered large quantities of the stems in spring and ate them at feasts. Haida women ate the shoots to purify their blood and make themselves beautiful. The more high-class Indians owned patches of evening primrose plants near their villages and anyone wanting to pick the stems had to ask permission to do so.

These plants were also used as a laxative (but never on an empty stomach), an astringent, in the form of poultices to help heal wounds and as an anti-scorbutic, a remedy for scurvy, a vitamin C deficiency disease.

The roots of the evening primrose plant, peeled and suitably cooked, were fed to convalescents. They were also made into a salve to help cure skin inflammations and eruptions. In addition, the bark and leaves of this incredibly versatile plant were used to relieve breathing difficulties, problems related to the stomach and intestines and to assuage certain female complaints.

Today, the roots are eaten in some countries, and the French use it to garnish salads. But it is the oil extracted from the plant's minuscule seeds that's the most wonderful of all. It is now being used systemically (pertaining to the whole body; internally) to treat many seemingly unrelated health disorders, and topically (pertaining to a definite area; externally) in the form of creams and lotions to moisturize, nourish, protect and beautify the skin.

Some say that the evening primrose plant originated in Mexico; others that it came from South America. But regardless of its origin, it now flourishes along the eastern seaboard of the USA and Canada, and thrives as well in Britain and Europe. In fact, it can be found on every continent and is actually being cultivated in many English gardens.

There was a time when the evening primrose plant was the focus of much attention and given the name of 'King's Cure All'. This appellation seemed appropriate, for the plant appeared most effective in relieving all sorts of ailments, including those of His Majesty himself. It then faded into temporary oblivion.

In 1970, scientists again explored, with renewed enthusiasm and excitement the potential of this seemingly amazing oil. Their experiments revealed that its *gamma-linolenic acid*, or GLA, was 10 times more biologically effective than linoleic acid.

One of the most eminently qualified and ardent researchers into the clinical and other applications of evening primrose oil is David Horrobin, MD, Ph.D.

Dr Horrobin, who had done impressive research into the role of PGE1 in schizophrenia, now began to consider its possible applications to a variety of other disorders. You may already be thinking: 'How can something used to treat a ''mental'' or personality disorder be applicable to the health of the skin, hair and nails?' The question would not be unreasonable if you don't see a connection. But there is, in fact, a link and it is that there's a common mechanism involved in a diverse number of disorders (e.g. skin inflammations, brittle nails, hair loss, blood vessel problems). What evening primrose oil seems to do is this: once in the body, its active principle (GLA) converts, without hindrance from multiple blocking agents, to PGE1. In other words, it's a precursor, or forerunner, of PGE1.

If you forget the meaning of terms used in this chapter you may wish to refresh your memory by glancing from time to time at Chapter 2, in which the EFA metabolic pathway is illustrated and described in detail. You may also find the glossary at the back of the book useful.

Efamol

Convinced, through diligent research, of the efficacy and potential of evening primrose oil as a unique source of PGE1, Dr Horrobin was instrumental in the founding of a company which would produce the oil according to the highest standards and market it. It was thus that Efamol Ltd came into being.

The seeds providing the oils used in the products *Efamol*, *Efavite* and the *Efamolia* range of skin care preparations are routinely analysed to ensure that there is no contamination and that the GLA content is according to strict specification. The oil itself is also routinely analysed.

What most appeals to some people working with and using *Efamol* is that it is a natural product, with no substantial adverse effects such as those produced by many medications and cosmetics on the market. It is therefore very compatible with nutritional approaches now increasingly adopted to deal safely, simply and effectively with a variety of troublesome conditions.

Generally, adults can use four *Efamol* capsules twice daily (half that for children), and a 6-week trial should tell you if treatment is going to be successful. Each capsule contains 500 mg (milligrams) evening primrose oil (45 mg GLA). The capsules may also be pierced and squeezed directly onto eczematous rashes, with beneficial results.

Noteworthy is the fact that three *Efamol* capsules contain as much GLA as a one-day supply of human breast milk, the only other truly reliable source of this very important nutrient.

5. WHAT YOUR HAIR, SKIN AND NAILS REVEAL

Skin is an indicator of our general health. All the body's living cells need oxygen and other forms of nourishment to thrive. When the diet is adequate and the blood circulation is able to carry oxygen effectively to every cell, the skin will show it. When these requisites are not met, skin problems arise and in perhaps no other instance is nutritional inadequacy as obvious as in abnormalities of the skin, hair and nails.

While most skin disorders are not life threatening, they can make our existence very uncomfortable. Since skin is that part of our body which we see and touch and which is visible to others, it plays a major role in how we feel and how we feel about ourselves. Consequently, it influences our willingness, or otherwise, to take part in social activities, and it affects our self-confidence.

Some skin problems respond well to simple treatments and minor changes in diet; others require medications and therapies best given or recommended by a medical doctor or dermatologist (skin specialist).

According to one physician, if remedies being tried for a particular problem seem to make it worse, stop them and consult a doctor (see Bibliography: Dvorine). *Check with your doctor*, too, if a condition shows no sign of improvement in about a week, except in cases of long-lasting disorders like acne, psoriasis and seborrhoea. With these, you may wish to give several different treatments a fair trial over, say, a 3- or 4-week period. Then, if there is no positive response, be sure to get professional help.

If your family doctor is unsure how to treat your problem, ask him or her to refer you to a dermatologist or other specialist, depending on the probable underlying cause or causes of the specific condition. In any case, if you are dissatisfied with the results of treatment, or with the doctor, do not hesitate to ask for a second opinion or even change doctors. It's *your* skin.

In Chapter 3, I mentioned several hair, skin and nail disorders related to a deficiency of certain vitamins, minerals and other nutrients. I shall now present additional information which will alert you to deviations from the normal condition of these structures. If you have any doubt at all as to what these abnormalities mean, particularly if they are coupled with other undesirable symptoms, do *consult a doctor*.

The Skin

Abnormal dryness may be due to impaired function of an endocrine gland called the thyroid, located in the neck. It may also suggest diabetes.

Acne is a temporary disturbance of the oil glands of the face, upper chest, upper back and shoulders. It is a common response to the hormonal changes of puberty. It appears when the sebaceous glands become clogged. Inflammation develops and bacteria ('germs') move in and cause infection. Blackheads and pimples may develop.

Treatment is best supervised by a dermatologist. It consists largely of instruction in cleansing the skin and advice on diet. Antibiotics may sometimes be prescribed. Acne is aggravated by stress, certain foods and some cosmetics.

The authors of *Doctor Zizmor's Guide to Clearer Skin* (see Bibliography) have described a form of acne which they have dubbed *working woman's acne*. It appears to be a response to the pressures of career life, especially when the woman has to divide her time among job, family and household chores.

Despite its name, though, working woman's acne is not the monopoly of the career woman working in a highly competitive environment. It is seen in fashion models with gruelling schedules and college and high school students with heavy work loads. It seems to be the skin's way of saying 'slow down!'

When trying to get rid of acne, points to remember are:

— Keep the hands away from the face as much as possible.
— Keep the scalp clean.
— Keep the hair clean and away from the face.
— Do not pick or squeeze pimples and blackheads.
  This can result in the spread of infection and more pimples.

Ashen coloration of the skin may be due to malignant disease, severe anaemia or kidney disease.

Bronzing is seen in Addinson's disease, in which the adrenal glands, located above the kidneys, are severely affected. It may also result from dyes or metals, and is an early sign of pellagra, which is caused by a deficiency of niacin (vitamin B_3).

Brownish-yellow spots, or 'liver spots', are sometimes seen in pregnancy, in diseases of the thyroid gland, malignant disease, sunburn, and as a reaction to some cosmetics.

Cherry-red skin is seen in carbon monoxide poisoning.

Cyanosis, in which the skin turns blue, is present in a wide range of disorders, including diseases of the heart and lungs.

Discolorations occur in conditions such as jaundice and malignant disease.

Eczema, or dermatitis, refers in general to inflammation of the skin. It is one of the most common skin disease. It is characterized by red, scaly, itching patches and can occur anywhere on the body, at any age. It indicates extreme sensitivity of the skin, and people with this condition are particularly vulnerable to temperature changes.

Before any treatment is started, it's best to determine the cause or causes, and the help of a doctor should be sought. Usually, creams or lotions are prescribed, but those containing anti-histamines or local anaesthetics should be avoided. Although somewhat effective in controlling the itching associated with eczema, these agents can actually lead to further itching as well as to inflammation.

Greasy ointments should also be avoided as they interfere with the evaporation of sweat and may increase itching. Be cautious, too, about lanolin. It seems to aggravate eczema in some persons. If you're one of these individuals, be sure to check for the presence of this ingredient in all soaps, cosmetics and other skin care products.

If you suspect that a certain food is contributing to your eczema, delete it from your diet. It can later be cautiously re-introduced. Despite the opinion of some doctors to the contrary, chocolate does seem to worsen the itching of eczematous conditions and is best omitted from the diet. Also avoid soft drinks.

A form of eczema commonly seen in homemakers, medical and nursing personnel and people in the food and drink trade is *housewives' eczema*, or 'dishpan hands'. It is also the most frequent dermatitis seen in industry.

Extra care should be taken to avoid irritating soaps, solvents, detergents, constant exposure to low humidity and over-washing of the hands. When rubber gloves are worn, it's best not to use hot water, which causes the hands to sweat and makes the eczema worse. Actually, vinyl gloves are better for handling potentially irritating substances.

Some vegetables, such as carrots, citrus fruits, garlic, onions, potatoes and tomatoes have been implicated in this skin condition. So have certain plants, metals and medications taken orally or applied to the skin.

There is another type of eczema called *atopic eczema*, to differentiate it from contact dermatitis, which is largely due to some irritant, for example a chemical or cosmetic.

A more precise term for this condition would be *atopic dermatitis*, according to Jon M. Hannifin, MD, an American dermatologist. This is because in older children and adults, the disorder is usually not eczematous — as it is in infants.

The word *atopy* comes from the Greek *atopia*, which means 'strangeness'. It is a word used clinically to refer to a group of diseases of an allergic nature. Atopic conditions differ from most allergies in that they seem to be inherited. The antibody produced, called atopic reagin or skin-sensitizing antibody, is deposited in the skin tissues and may enter the blood-stream.

Factors that seem to trigger atopic dermatitis include skin irritants, too much heat, over-exertion and sweating, allergens (substances producing allergy), infection and emotional stress. In fact, emotional stress is perhaps the most potent trigger factor for atopic dermatitis.

The primary reaction that occurs is a type of swelling, such as is seen in hay fever or inflammation of the nasal passages. The chief symptoms are asthma, inflamed nostrils and urticaria, characterized by itchy bumps on the skin.

A recent study showed that three weeks' treatment with *Efamol* evening primrose oil, taken internally, produced a small but significant improvement in patients with atopic dermatitis.

Earlier experiments revealed that children with atopic dermatitis have a decreased level of unsaturated fatty acids in the blood, and one study has shown that treatment with linoleic acid and gamma-linolenic acid (GLA), in the form of *Efamol* evening primrose oil, improves the symptoms of atopic dermatitis by approximately 30 per cent.

One other thing about persons with atopic dermatitis: there appears to be a defect in the function of the enzyme delta-6-desaturase (D6D), which leads to an accumulation of linoleic acid and a lack of all further products on the metabolic pathway (see Chapter 2).

Efamol contains GLA, which can bypass this suspected enzyme defect and bring about an improvement in the condition. At the same time, it helps to shift the whole biochemical pattern toward normality.

Psoriasis is a chronic, recurring, non-contagious skin condition that is thought to be genetically determined. It can occur at any age. It is characterized by sharply defined patches of scales which can occur anywhere in the body.

Although the cause of the condition is said to be unknown, positive response to treatment with evening primrose oil in some individuals suggests an underlying deficiency as a contributing factor.

The course of the disorder is affected by injury, infection, stress and drugs. One co-worker told me that, in the 1970s, she knew several women who developed psoriasis following general anaesthetic and the use of certain medications.

Rash is a general word applied to any eruption, or 'breaking out', of the skin, especially in association with contagious diseases. It is also one of the most common side effects of a number of medications, a fact that seems to have eluded many doctors' consciousness.

In my work at the hospital I see many cases of skin rash and my first reaction is to check the medications the affected patients are taking. After that, I review their diets. In most cases, I would say, the rashes are drug and diet related.

Rashes are usually red or pink in colour and temporary only. Here are some types of rash you may encounter:

Nappy rash: inflammation of the skin of infants, in the nappy area, usually due to an irritant.

Heat rash, or miliaria, is caused by the obstruction of sweat gland ducts. It is most commonly seen in infants, obese persons and individuals exposed to excessive heat for prolonged periods.

Associated with heat rash is a condition called *hyperhidrosis* (excessive sweating). It is a functional overactivity of the sweat glands caused by certain fevers and stimulants, and sometimes by migraine.

Nettle rash (hives or *urticaria*) is thought to be due to an allergic substance or food, and in some persons to heat or cold. More commonly though, urticaria is caused by medications. Almost any drug can be responsible — medications for colds; suppositories for haemorrhoids (piles); contraceptive pills. But antibiotics, sedatives, tranquillizers, analgesics ('pain-killers'), diuretics and laxatives are among the worst culprits.

All medications, including those purchased without prescription, should be regarded as potential causes of urticaria. If you don't absolutely need them, do without them.

All urticaria sufferers should be screened for collagen, blood vessel, infectious and malignant diseases.

Wrinkling of the skin, if permanent, may be a result of ageing. If temporary, it may be due to prolonged immersion in water or to dehydration. (For more information on wrinkling, see Chapters 1 and 9.)

Yellow skin is usually a sign of jaundice or liver disorder.

The Hair

One of the greatest concerns many men have, and now an increasing number of women, is abnormal hair loss, or *alopecia*.

Here are some types of alopecia, which will subsequently be indicated by the letter 'A'.

A. adnata:	congenital baldness, or baldness at birth
A. areata:	well-defined patches of baldness, which leave the scalp smooth and white; patchy baldness
A. follicularis:	hair loss due to inflammation of hair follicles
A. neurotica:	baldness following a nervous disorder or injury to the nervous system
A. senilis:	the baldness of old age
A. symptomatica:	hair loss following prolonged fevers, or from changes in internal secretions
A. toxica:	hair loss due to poisons from infectious diseases

Other causes of abnormal hair loss in general include hereditary factors, impaired blood circulation, stress, the ageing process, certain illnesses and infections, imbalance of hormones, nervous disorders and injury to the nervous system toxic substances including drugs, general ill health and dietary deficiencies.

Dandruff

Dandruff, or *seborrhoea*, is a functional disease of the sebaceous, or oil-secreting, glands of the skin, which of course includes the scalp.

These glands are located in the second layer of scalp tissue and are usually linked to the hair follicle. They secrete *sebum*, an oily substance which helps to keep the hair resilient.

Seborrhoea is characterized by an increased amount, and sometimes altered quality, of sebum. The production of sebum is influenced by diet, the building up and breaking down process of tissue cells (metabolism), emotional factors, endocrine gland function and blood circulation.

Excessive dandruff is one of the main contributing causes of abnormal hair loss, and the bulk of available evidence suggests that it is caused by chemical reactions occurring inside the body. These reactions, it appears, are largely influenced by faulty diet, stress and unintelligent use of hair care products.

The small whitish flakes characteristic of dandruff are unmistakable. They can appear in and behind the ears as well as on the scalp. Their presence on the clothing can ruin otherwise impeccable grooming and create a bad impression. Suggestions for controlling and treating this irritating condition are given in Chapter 8.

The Nails

Both the function and appearance of the nails may be influenced by a number of factors, including infections, tumours, medical conditions and changes associated with some skin disorders.

Changes in the nails, such as ridges and white spots, often signal nutritional deficiencies (see Chapter 3). Here are other clues nails give as to our state of health.

Curving of the nails is seen in some heart and lung conditions and can be excessive. It is sometimes coupled with club-shaped fingers.

Discolorations

Black nails are sometimes seen in diabetes and other forms of gangrene. Any persisting black coloration should be promptly checked by a doctor.

Blue-black nails are common and are usually due to bleeding and bleeding diseases such as haemophilia, as well as to injury.

Blueness (cyanosis) of the nails usually indicates anaemia, poor blood circulation or injury. Some chemicals stain the nails blue. Check with your doctor to rule out malignancy.

Brown nails can indicate arsenic poisoning.

Brownish-black nails are a sign of chronic mercurial poisoning.

Green nails can result from contact with some chemicals, but they may also indicate internal disease or a reaction to certain drugs.

Slate-coloured nails are an early sign of the over-administration of silver (argyria), and treatment should be stopped immediately. Years ago, some nose and eye drops contained silver.

Dry, malformed nails may be signs of nerve injury; or Raynaud's disease, which is caused by spasm of blood vessels of he extremities, or of syphilis or other health disorders.

Eggshell nails, in which the nails are soft and transparent, bend easily and split at the ends, are associated with arthritis, nerve inflammations and leprosy, and may be the only visible indication of late syphilis.

Fragile nails that split often may be the result of prolonged contact with chemicals or to manicuring too frequently.

Hard, brittle nails may indicate gout and other related metabolic disorders. Brittleness and even separation of nails can occur in pregnancy, as well as after giving birth if the woman is breast-feeding. This is because the mother's body is diverting protein and other essential nutrients to the baby. A healthy diet is therefore vital.

Ingrown toenails may be a reminder that you are not cutting the nails properly, or that you're wearing poorly fitting shoes which place undue pressure on the edges of the nails.

Longitudinal striations, or stripes, seen on the nails of persons past middle life, are associated with *onchorrhexis,* an abnormal brittleness and splitting of the nails.

These signs may be clues to a possible focus of infection, for example in the bowel or at the root of a tooth, and should be promptly investigated.

Lack of certain nutrients in the diet is also a possible cause, and in Chapter 10 you will read of one such deficiency and of its successful correction, with consequent healing of the nails.

Pitted nails, in which there are minute depressions, are often associated with psoriasis. They are also sometimes seen in people with alopecia areata (see section on the hair).

Racquet nails, which are flat and cross-hatched like the strings of a tennis racquet, sometimes result from habitually biting and sucking the thumb.

Spoon-shaped nails, which are depressed in the centre, may be a sign of a type of anaemia, heart disease, or achlorhydria, a condition in which free hydrochloric acid is absent from the stomach. They could also be the result of long-term use of strong soaps or solvents.

Transverse, or Beau's lines may appear following damage to the nail bed. The approximate date of the damage can be determined, since it takes four to six months for the nail to grow. Transverse ridges are sometimes formed during menstruation. They are also sometimes seen in some women after childbirth. Usually the nails revert to normal over a period of months, as the ridges grow out and new, healthy nail grows in.

White spots. Striped spots, more frequent in women than in men, may be due to injury. Transverse white bands in all nails may indicate arsenic poisoning. Other white spots are usually signs of a zinc deficiency.

Yellow nails may signal a blood disorder, or they may be the result of contact with certain chemicals.

The foregoing information should be regarded as a guide to possible underlying causes or contributing factors in abnormalities of the skin, hair and nails. It is not intended as a substitute for a doctor's diagnosis or medical treatment.

It is well to remember, too, that each of us is a unique individual. What may be a symptom or sign of a particular disorder for one person may be due to an entirely different cause in another.

6. How Stress Affects Hair, Skin And Nails

Stress occurs when the demands of our environment tax or overwhelm our personal resources to deal with them. These demands can be external, as in the work place or in a social setting, or they can originate from within ourselves.

We cannot live without some stress. It is what propels some of us toward achievement. It is when stress is ongoing and unrelieved that it becomes a destructive force. We see striking evidence of its damage in some forms of heart disease, for example. We also see its deleterious effects in certain skin conditions, in damaged nails and in falling hair. In some forms of dermatitis, for instance, there is a strong stress component.

Stressors
A stressor is something that causes stress or leads to it. Infamous stressors include uncertainty, anxiety, frustration, conflict and failure. Too many life change events occurring in too short a space of time also generate stress. So do emotions suppressed rather than expressed.

Stress is usually in the eye of the beholder. What may be stressful for one person may be a challenge or pleasant stimulus for another. It's how we view an event or circumstance that determines whether or not it will be a source of stress for us.

Stress and tension
Many people think of stress and tension as the same thing. Tension, though, is only one symptom of stress. It occurs when our muscles over-contract, or tighten unduly. When this happens,

unnecessary pressure is exerted on underlying structures such as nerves and blood vessels, preventing them from functioning properly. We then experience a number of unpleasant sensations which include aches, pain, itching and cold hands and feet.

Body changes during stress

In times of stress, certain changes occur in the functioning of the body's internal structures, under hormonal influence. These include:

— a rise in blood-pressure;

— a constricting, or narrowing, of blood vessels at the body's extremities, e.g. the hands, feet and scalp;

— retention of salt, and consequently of fluids, in the tissues;

— heightened stimulation of nerve endings, e.g. in the skin;

— skin changes, e.g. 'goose bumps' and 'hair standing on end'.

Stress-related disorders

Probably more than 50 per cent of all diseases are stress related. Noteworthy among these are arthritis, asthma, bronchitis, cancer and heart disease. But there are others which, if not as incapacitating or life threatening, are nevertheless uncomfortable and detract substantially from the joy of living.

Stress and the skin

One of these stress related disorders is the skin rash called eczema. It has been linked to frustration — a powerful stressor. I know someone who has gone from doctor to doctor for treatment for a skin rash, with no success. Finally, a specialist to whom she was referred helped her to identify an underlying psychological factor contributing to the rash, and the associated itching that was driving her almost crazy. It was frustration with her two teenagers, with whom she was unable to communicate satisfactorily. With the help of the counsellor, she changed her strategy in dealing with the youngsters, and relationships improved markedly. With her sense of inadequacy and her frustration gone, her rash quickly cleared up with medication.

When I was about 20 years old, I was attracted to a young man whom my mother regarded as most unsuitable for me. She did everything in her power to discourage me from seeing him and him from seeing me. I became deeply distressed. I developed on my face what appeared to be a sunburn and when people mistook it for such and commented on it accordingly, I did not disillusion them. But I knew only too well that it was not the sun's rays that had altered my skin. I realized even then, that it was the suppression of the anguish and frustration I was experiencing that had brought about my skin disorder.

Fortunately, the emotional problem resolved itself, and my skin regained its previous attractive qualities as dramatically as it had deteriorated, without any medical intervention whatever.

We know that adrenalin is released into the system during stressful situations, often called times of 'fight or flight', such as when we feel threatened. There is yet another hormone, secreted when threats are not as obvious or identifiable as, say, when someone is about to deal us a physical blow. It is called *serotonin*. It is a potent vasoconstrictor, that is, it causes blood vessels to narrow so that blood flow is restricted. Interestingly, it has been found in cancerous tumours. Serotonin seems to be produced during emotional stress and to aggravate anxiety and other nervous states. One doctor has referred to it as 'the ultimate downer'.

So even though we may have succeeded in fooling others by 'putting up a front', we cannot possibly deceive our body. Our internal states have a profound effect on our external conditions. This is partially because the muscles and skin forming the outer covering of our body have a close connection, through the nervous system, with inside structures. Feelings such as rage and frustration disturb the harmonious functioning of the endocrine, nervous and blood circulatory systems. When these systems are upset, we see and feel the results. The condition of the hair, skin and nails is sometimes the first clue as to this dysfunction.

Stress and the hair

Scientific literature on this subject abounds with persuasive evidence of the stress–tension–baldness relationship. As early as

1900, researchers suggested that scalp tension was a factor contributing to common baldness in humans. Others found that women and children, who had thicker and looser scalp tissues than men, did not have the problem of balding male adults did.

Yet another researcher removed elliptical segments of scalp tissue from monkeys and then stitched together the remaining skin edges to form a tighter scalp. A persisting baldness, such as is seen in humans, resulted. Obviously, increased scalp tension and the consequent heightened pressure on underlying blood vessels impeded nourishment to the cells of the scalp tissue.

Even facial tension has been implicated in abnormal hair loss. Two University of Chicago psychiatrists found that facial tension leads to increased scalp tension which in turn compresses structures vital to the flourishing of the hair.

The consensus of experts is that the structures primarily involved in the thriving of the hair are the circulatory and endocrine systems. Both can be influenced by exercise and relaxation.

In the previous section, I related how my skin had changed in response to stress. At that same time, my hair also suffered. It began to fall out at an alarming rate. A cousin, at whose house I was spending a day and who had noted the heavy hair fall in the bathtub, remarked that she had never seen anyone lose so much hair at any one time. Happily, as occurred with my skin, the condition of my hair improved when the cause of my emotional upheaval ceased to exist. My hair once again became shiny and luxuriant.

Stress and the nails
During stressful situations, one of the changes occurring is the dilation, or widening, of blood vessels supplying vital organs and the constriction, or narrowing, of structures at the body's extremities. That is why some people's hands and feet are cold when they are under stress and therefore tense. As they relax, the hands and feet become warm.

It is therefore not difficult to appreciate how stress, particularly if prolonged and unmitigated, can adversely affect the nails. Because of diminished blood flow to the fingers and toes, nutrients to these parts are undersupplied and deficiencies become manifest. Among the signs of such deficiencies are nails that are brittle and which peel, split or break easily or develop white spots.

Stress can influence the rate at which nails grow. Nail biting, a practice in which some persons indulge when under stress, can almost double the rate of nail growth. This is a compensatory activity in which the epithelium responds to mechanical stress or injury. A similar accelerated rate of nail growth is seen as a result of some occupational stresses.

Dealing with stress

Stress is largely a matter of individual perception. Coping with stress depends, to a great extent, on one's personal attitudes toward it and one's resources for dealing with it.

Most authorities on the subject, however, suggest a number of coping strategies that can be useful to everyone, provided that an honest effort is made to apply them. Here are a few you might like to consider.

— Try to avoid too many life change events in any one year. For example, if you have just ended a close relationship, it's probably not a good idea to change jobs, sell your house and enter into another relationship all in the same year. Give yourself time and be patient.

— Whether working or playing, try to avoid great contrasts in levels of activity, as a general rule. Try to establish a certain evenness of the pace of living without generating boredom, which is itself stressful.

— Learn to listen to, and heed, your body's cues. For this, you need to set aside a short period every day for some form of relaxation or meditation to quieten your mind and replenish your reserves. I have given a specimen meditation later in this chapter.

— To avoid overcommitment — in which you end up having too many things to do and not enough time in which to do them all satisfactorily — learn to say 'no' when this is appropriate.

In stress management classes which I have instructed in my community, most participants said they found this one of the hardest things to do. They either didn't try to do it in order to avoid 'making waves', as they put it, or if they did try to do it they ended up feeling guilty.

The March/April 1986 issue of *Health League News Digest* offers these tips on the subject:

— You, too, have rights. You, too, are important.

— Realizing your own needs doesn't mean that you are insensitive to the needs of others.

— Be assertive. Maintain eye contact when saying 'no' to someone, and speak clearly.

— You may have to repeat yourself. You may have, for example, to say: 'No, I'm sorry I can't do that right now. I will do it when I can.'

— Be honest about your feelings. Express them. If you don't, they will turn inward and cause you harm by adversely affecting *your* health.

Assertiveness, self-confidence and self-respect can help to eliminate feelings of guilt which often accompany having to say 'no'. They are habits worth developing.

Meditating

The best definition of 'meditation' I've yet seen is that of Dr Lawrence LeShan, author of *How to Meditate* (see Bibliography). Dr LeShan describes meditation as doing one thing, and only one thing, at a time. Attention is focused intently on one object or activity at a time to the exclusion of everything else that's unrelated. It doesn't only mean sitting cross-legged and reiterating a prescribed mantra (word or phrase).

Among the benefits derived from regular meditation are a deeply relaxed physiological (referring to body function) state, with an accompanying alertness of the mind; lower metabolic rate; lowered blood-pressure and increased skin resistance indicating decreased anxiety and tension.

What all this means, in essence, is that the signals the body receives and to which it responds during meditation are simpler and more coherent than at almost any other time.

Increasingly, doctors are recommending meditation for a variety of health disorders. For your own reassurance, however, do *obtain your doctor's permission* to practise the specimen meditation that follows.

Before meditating

— Choose a quiet place where you are unlikelyto be disturbed for 10 to 20 minutes.

— Sit comfortably and naturally erect. Support your head and spine if necessary. Relax your hands. Relax the rest of your body. Close your eyes.

— Let go of tightness in your jaws by unclenching your teeth. Breathe slowly, smoothly and naturally.

The Meditation

1. Inhale normally through your nostrils.
2. Exhale through the nostrils and mentally count 'one'.
3. Inhale again, as before.
4. Exhale and mentally count 'two'.
5. Repeat steps 1 to 4, mentally counting 'three' and 'four' with the third and fourth *exhalations*.
6. Repeat steps 1 to 5, again and again, until your predetermined meditation time is up.
7. Open your eyes, leisurely stretch your limbs and unhurriedly prepare to resume your other activities.

N.B. While doing your meditation, you may find that your thoughts stray to other things than the awareness of your breathing and the counting of your respirations. Don't worry about this. It is normal, especially for beginning meditators. Simply guide your attention back to your meditation and start all over again. For best results, persevere.

The Curling Leaf

Here's a little exercise — actually more of a posture than an exercise — that is very effective in promoting total relaxation.

It encourages a rich supply of blood to the neck, face and scalp, and because it reduces tension that has accumulated in the whole body, it improves the circulation to the hands and feet, thereby benefiting the nails.

How to do it
1. Sit upright on your heels, Japanese style.
2. Slowly bend forward and gently rest your forehead on the mat, or turn your head to the side if this is more comfortable. Relax your arms and hands beside you, with your palms turned upward (Figure 4).

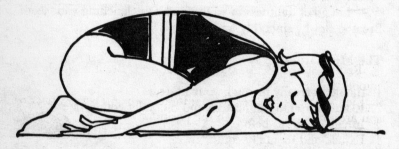

Figure 4: The Curling Leaf

3. Remain in this position as long as you're comfortable in it, breathing naturally.
4. Slowly sit up.

Legs Up
Here's another posture you can use as an alternative to *The Shoulderstand*, described in Chapter 7.

It relaxes tired feet and legs and reduces any swelling present; discourages the formation of varicose veins and beautifies the legs; promotes relaxation of the whole body and thereby contributes to healthy-looking skin all over.

How to do it
1. Lie on your mat near a wall and rest your feet against it (Figure

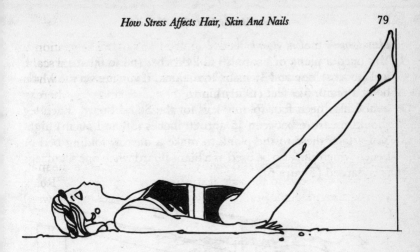

Figure 5: Legs Up

5). Relax your arms and hands beside you. Breathe slowly and smoothly.

2. Lie like this for at least three minutes to begin with; longer as you are more comfortable in the position.

3. To come out of the posture, bend your legs and bring your knees toward your chest. Roll onto your side and use your hands to help you up.

The Slant Board

Unless you have high blood-pressure or a heart or breathing disorder, here's a health and beauty aid worth investing in. But first, *check with your doctor* before making use of it.

Called the Slant Board, it allows you to lie in a hips-high, head-low position similar to that achieved when practising *The Shoulderstand*, described in Chapter 7, but without the effort. The benefits it produces with regular use are similar to those obtained through faithful practice of the Shoulderstand.

You can buy a Slant Board from some department stores, health food stores or medical supply houses. You can also prop the tapered end of an ironing board on a sturdy piece of furniture. Or you can make your own.

How to make a Slant Board

You need a plank of board 20 to 24 inches (50 to 60cm) wide, 6 feet (180cm) long and ¾ inch (2cm) thick. If you are very tall, you need a plank 6½ feet (195cm) long.

You also need four folding legs for the Sland Board. Each leg should measure between 15 and 20 inches (38 and 50cm) high. You attach these to the plank to make a narrow folding bed or bench which can also be used as a Slant Board when one set of legs is collapsed (Figure 6).

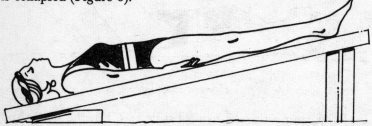

Figure 6: The Slant Board

You may cover your Slant Board with foam about 3 inches (7.5cm) thick and fabric of your choice.

To use the Slant Board

Lie with your head at the lower end of the board, as in the illustration. If you wish, you may put a small, soft pillow or cushion under your head.

This is an excellent time to apply a good quality moisturizing cream to your face. Choose one that's rich in nutrients, such as the type of skin care products mentioned in Chapter 9. As you lie on the Slant Board, increasingly relaxed, the beneficial substances in the cream or lotion will be absorbed into your system to nourish and beautify your skin.

Close your eyes. Breathe slowly, smoothly and rhythmically. With each exhalation, imagine breathing away fatigue and cares. As you lie there, visualize the little lines of worry and tiredness on your face fading away. Mentally picture your features becoming softer, gentler and more youthful. Lie there for 10 to 20 minutes, savouring the tranquility that will enfold and rejuvenate you.

After your allotted time on the Slant Board, open your eyes and slowly and carefully get up. Stretch leisurely from top to toe and luxuriate in the feeling of well-being you experience.

7. Exercises For Healthy Hair, Skin And Nails

The collagen and elastic fibres found in the dermis are responsible for the toughness and elasticity of your skin. The loss of subcutaneous fat (under the dermis layer), the decrease in the number of elastic fibres and some loss of muscle tone all contribute to premature wrinkling and sagging of the skin. This process can start as early as in the twenties.

Blood circulation
We know that every single cell of the body depends on an adequate supply of healthy blood for nourishment and renewal. If you multiply the number of cells found in one square inch (6 square centimetres) of skin by the amount of skin in your body, you will quickly appreciate the vital importance of an adequate, unobstructed blood circulation. In the case of the skin on the head — the scalp — the blood has to travel 'uphill' as it were, and not infrequently reaches its destination substantially diminished. Abnormal hair loss is only one consequence of this deprivation.

The lymphatic system
Our blood circulation is intimately connected to our lymphatic system, an important function of which is to eliminate germs and poisons from the body.

Lymph is the tissue fluid that bathes all our cells. It is similar to the liquid part of blood (plasma) but it contains less protein. Unlike plasma, however, lymph contains no red blood cells. Lymph provides nourishment and oxygen to tissue cells and carries wastes away from them.

The endocrine glands

The blood circulation also works closely with the endocrine glands which pour out their secretions directly into the blood-stream. Every single cell is under endocrine gland control. The pituitary, located in the brain, and no bigger than a pea, is the master gland which controls the function of all the other endocrine glands. The thyroid, found in the neck, regulates metabolism, and the adrenals, situated above the kidneys, play a crucial part in stress reactions.

Working together

These three systems — the blood circulatory, lymphatic and endocrine — are in turn intimately linked to the nervous system, and the four have a close collaboration in maintaining the health of all cells, tissues and organs.

You will recall that when we were in the embryonic stages of our development, hair, skin, nails and nervous system shared a common tissue. Since the skin is the largest organ, it is therefore not difficult to see how enormously it can be affected by a breakdown in the harmonious functioning of these vital systems.

Value of exercise

Skin, like any other body structure, atrophies (wastes away) with inactivity. For skin to be taut and smooth and glow with health, regular exercise is imperative.

I've watched, with fascination, the young-looking fingers of the elderly world-renowned classical guitarist, the late Andres Segovia, and saw in them evidence of this statement. I've also marvelled at the youthful hands of the well-known American violinist, Itzhak Perlman, as his fingers glided effortlessly along the strings of his instrument. I felt sure that they were partially the result of years of constant exercise.

Apart from the special selection of exercises offered in this chapter, I urge you to engage in regular outdoor activity compatible with your state of health, your lifestyle and weather conditions. Possibilities range from brisk walking, bicycling, tennis, cross-country skiing or any other aerobic type of exercise you enjoy. It is important to choose something that you *will do* and which you find pleasurable, rather than something that is currently in vogue, so as not to generate distress (harmful stress) which will rob your skin of its radiance and other youthful qualities.

Exercise and the lymphatic system

When muscles contract during exercise, they exert pressure on lymphatic vessels. This stimulates the flow of lymph through the body and promotes effective elimination of waste matter.

The exercises presented in this chapter enhance lymph circulation in at least three ways:

(1) By stimulation, through a gentle massage action when muscles press against large blood vessels (arteries), which in turn exert gentle pressure on lymphatic vessels.

(2) By stretching, which temporarily removes 'kinks' from the lymphatic vessels, making the flow of lymph much smoother. In the upside-down exercises (e.g., *The Shoulderstand*), the lymphatic vessels are afforded a rest, since lymph now travels downward rather than on its usual uphill course.

(3) By improving the tone of muscles and underlying blood and lymphatic vessels, through gentle stretching movements and sustained stretches.

A healthier lymphatic system results in more effective elimination of surplus fluid, toxins and other undesirable products from the body. The consequence is better overall health and appearance. Firm, clear skin, abundant, shiny hair and strong beautiful nails are unmistakable signs of radiant health.

Other benefits

Apart from their benefits to the lymphatic system, the exercises to follow have been thoughtfully chosen because of their special benefits to the blood circulatory, endocrine and nervous systems, and through them to the hair, skin and nails. They have also been selected because they help improve and preserve good muscle tone and mass and the quality of the supporting subcutaneous tissues.

The exercises offered in this chapter have the added benefit of promoting relaxation by reducing the build-up of unnecessary tension. Tension build up is one of the most destructive forces to affect the human organism adversely, and therefore also the integrity of the hair, skin and nails.

Preparing for the exercises

- *Ask your doctor* if you may practise these exercises.
- Practise faithfully, at about the same time each day, or *at least every other day*. Ten minutes practice a day are worth more than one hour once a week only.
- Practise on an empty or near-empty stomach; never immediately after a meal.
- Be comfortable. Empty your bladder and bowel and wear loose-fitting garments that allow you to move, stretch and breathe freely.
- Be safe. Remove from your person all sharp objects, such as pens, pencils and hairpins.
- *Always warm up first*, to avoid muscular pulls and strains.
- Practise on a firm, well-padded surface, such as a carpet or folded blankets on the floor. I shall refer to this surface as the 'mat'.

Warm-ups

The neck.

1. Sit naturally erect with your hands relaxed in your lap. Close your eyes if you wish. Breathe normally throughout the exercises.
2. Imagine a large figure-eight lying on its side, in front of you. Slowly and smoothly trace its outline with your nose, three or four times.
3. Repeat step 2 in the other direction.
4. Rest.

Also for the neck.

1. Sit naturally erect with your hands relaxed. Close your eyes if you wish, and remember to keep breathing naturally.

2. Keeping shoulders and arms relaxed, tilt your head sideways, aiming your left ear toward your left shoulder.
3. Bring your head upright.
4. Now tilt your right ear toward your right shoulder.
5. Bring your head upright.
6. Repeat steps 2 to 5 three or four times, slowly, smoothly and with complete awareness.

These neck warm-ups tone and firm the muscles that run from below the ears, across the neck and into the chest. They also exercise the *platysma*, a flat muscle lying beneath the skin, which maintains the contour of the neck. They improve the blood circulation to the face and scalp and are useful for reducing tension built up in the neck.

The shoulders.
1. Sit naturally upright on your mat. Relax your arms and hands. Breathe normally.
2. Slowly and smoothly circle your shoulders with a forward-to-backward motion, three or four times. Rest.
3. Repeat step 2 in the opposite direction. Rest.

This warm-up enhances the effects of the neck exercises just described. It improves the blood circulation to the upper body and reduces the build-up of tension in the shoulders and upper back.

An all-over warm-up.
1. Sit naturally upright, with your legs bent and soles flat on your mat, close to your bottom.
2. Pass your arms *under* your bent knees and hug your thighs close to you. Curve your back as much as possible and tuck your chin down. Maintain this curved position throughout the exercise and keep breathing naturally.
3. Roll onto your back; kick backward.
4. Kick forward to come up again, lightly on your feet so as not to jar your spine.
5. Repeat steps 3 and 4, in smooth succession, as many times as you wish.
6. Rest.

This warm-up improves the blood circulation in the spine and benefits the many nerves branching off it. It warms up the whole body and gives a feeling of exhilaration. It is sometimes called the *Rock-and-roll*.

The Exercises

For the face and scalp

I'm not keen on most of the facial exercises I've seen described and illustrated in various beauty books. I tend to agree with Albert M. Kligman, director of the Aging Skin Clinic of the Hospital of the University of Pennsylvania in Philadelphia, USA. Dr Kligman believes that special facial exercises promote wrinkling. The muscles of your face, he remarks, are designed essentially to open and close your mouth and eyes, so usually get plenty of exercise.

There is, however, one exercise that I consider excellent. It's called *The Lion*, and I like it for these reasons.

— It reduces tension in the jaws. Dentists will tell you that most people have tight jaws. This leads to headaches which, like other forms of pain, can in time etch disfiguring marks on the face.

— It improves the tone of the neck muscles, helps to improve the voice — and therefore the personality — and relieves a sore throat.

— It encourages a rich supply of blood to the face and scalp and in this respect is a natural beautifier.

How to do it.

1. Sit naturally upright on your mat, with hands relaxed. Breathe normally.
2. *Exhaling*, stick out your tongue as far as comfortable with jaws open as widely as possible.
3. At the same time, stare as fiercely as you can. Tense all facial muscles (Figure 7).
4. Exhalation complete, inhale, close your jaws and eyes and relax all muscles. Imagine all tension draining away. Visualize the little lines of fatigue on your face fading and your features becoming softer and more serene.

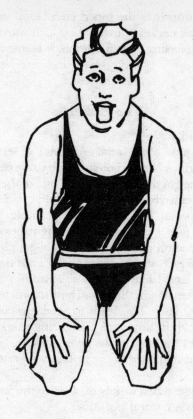

Figure 7: The Lion

For the hands

This exercise, known as *The Flower*, is excellent for improving the blood circulation to the hands and fingernails. It helps keep the fingers supple, graceful and young looking, and prevents the accumulation of tension in the hands.

How to do it.

1. Sit naturally upright on your mat.
2. Hold your hands, made into tight fists, in front of you. (*Do not*

simultaneously clench your teeth; keep your jaws relaxed and breathe naturally.)

3. Open your hands *very slowly and with resistance*. It may help you to think of them as tightly closed, sleeping buds, unwillingly opening to the sun's rays (Figure 8).

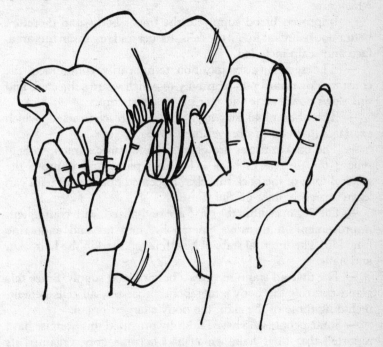

Figure 8: The Flower

4. When your hands are fully open, give the fingers a final stretch until they arch backward. Then stretch the arms sideways, as far as they will go, and hold the open-arms position for a few seconds.

5. Repeat the exercise once or twice.

6. Relax your arms and hands.

7. If you wish, you may add to this exercise by vigorously shaking your hands, as if ridding them of drops of water, until they tingle.

For the whole body

Here's an exercise, deservedly called 'the queen of exercises'. Do *ask your doctor* if you can practise it, especially if you suffer from a heart or lung condition or have high blood-pressure. Called *The Shoulderstand*, this exercise has far-reaching health benefits, some of which are:

— Improved blood supply to the upper body, and therefore better nourishment for all the cells, tissues and organs in this area, face and scalp included.

— The semi-inverted position temporarily counteracts the constant downward pull of gravity to which we're subjected, and this slows down wear and tear on vital structures.

— The abdominal and neck muscles are contracted, which exercises them and improves their tone.

— The back muscles are given a therapeutic stretch, to help relieve the distress of back aches and pains and improve the general tone of the back muscles. Repeated episodes of pain can leave unsightly lines on the features.

— The organs within the torso are revitalized, with consequent improvement in digestive, metabolic, nervous and endocrine function. The internal state of health is reflected in the hair, skin and nails.

— The thyroid gland receives a better blood supply. Since this gland controls the body's metabolic processes, all cells benefit, including those of the skin, the body's largest organ.

— Some people who have faithfully practised this exercise have reported that their hair, which had become grey, regained its original colour.

How to do it.

1. Lie on your back on a mat. Bend your knees and rest your soles flat on the mat. Place your arms close beside you.
2. Bring first one knee then the other to the chest.
3. Straighten one leg at a time until the feet point upward.
4. Kick backward with both feet until the hips are clear of the mat. Support the hips with the hands, thumbs in front (Figure 9).
5. Maintain this head-low, hips-high position for, say 10 seconds

to begin with, breathing normally. As you become more accustomed to the posture, hold it longer, working up to 3 or more minutes.

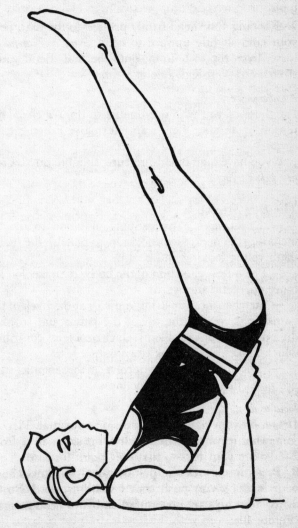

Figure 9: The Shoulderstand

To come out of position

6. Concentrate so as to maintain your balance as you remove your hands from your hips and rest them on the mat, close to your body.

7. Keeping your head firmly pressed to the mat, perhaps tilting your chin slightly upward to help, *slowly and carefully* lower your torso, from top to bottom, onto the mat. Bend your knees and stretch out your legs, one at a time.

An alternative

For those of you who are unable to do *The Shoulderstand* for one reason or another, here's an alternative exercise called *The Dog Stretch*.

If you have high blood-pressure, though, do *check with your doctor first before trying it.*

The Dog Stretch

— Encourages a rich supply of blood to the upper body, including the neck, face and scalp, to nourish the tissues and keep them young looking and healthy.

— Promotes relaxation of the body, to make you look and feel more energetic afterwards.

— Stetches the hamstring muscles at the back of the legs. The hamstrings control the tilt of the pelvis and so play a part in discouraging back problems. Back problems contribute to stress, which makes people look worn-out.

— The arms and legs receive a therapeutic stretch, which promotes firmness and shapeliness.

How to do it.

1. Get on your hands and knees on your mat. Place your hands somewhat forward so that your arms slope away from you.

2. Tuck in your toes so that they point forward.

3. Pressing on toes and palms, raise your knees and straighten your legs. *Carefully* push your heels downward. Straighten your arms. Your hips are now raised and your head hangs downward. (Figure 10).

4. Maintain this position for 5 to 10 seconds to start with,

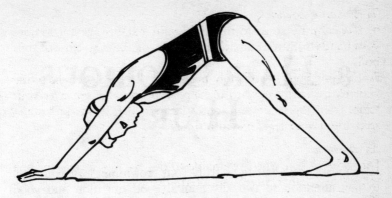

Figure 10: The Dog Stretch

breathing normally. As you become more comfortable with the posture, hold it for a minute or more.

To come out of position.
5. Gently rock forward, lower your knees to the mat and point the toes backward.

Sit on your heels or in another comfortable position and rest.

8. HAIR GLORIOUS HAIR

If you want your hair to be truly your crowning glory, you need to pay attention to two key points: good nutrition and good hygiene. Remember that scalp is skin, and hair is a modified form of skin, and both require the same nutrients for optimum health.

Hygiene

Authorities on hair care emphasize the importance of good scalp and hair hygiene for keeping hair on the head and for keeping it healthy and looking good. They say that often, proper hygiene, faithfully carried out, helps to control abnormal hair loss. They add that, without good hygiene habits, no treatment for slowing down hair loss and maintaining healthy hair can be effective.

Before shampooing

Like skin elsewhere on the body, the scalp provides a waterproof covering. Nevertheless, it contains tiny openings — pores — which permit some absorption of topical (local) applications. These, sensibly chosen and used, can complement substances used systemically.

Although many commercial hair care products are harsh and potentially harmful, some contain natural ingredients which benefit scalp and hair. Look on labels for the inclusion of substances from natural sources, such as aloe vera, apricot kernel oil, biotin (one of the B vitamins) camomile, henna, jojoba, marshmallow and nettle leaves, peach kernels or buds, pepper grass, rosemary, sea kelp, wheatgerm, willow leaves and bark and vitamins.

Scalp massage

According to Philip Kingsley, an internationally known trichologist, head massage is one of the exercises you must do each day as part of your complete programme to maintain a healthy scalp and healthy hair.

Benefits.

Scalp massage brings extra blood to the tissues, which helps to enhance the delivery of nutrients, oxygen and hormones to hair follicles. It also reduces scalp tension, which can contribute to hair loss. In fact, some experts on hair care consider that the first essential in treating hair problems is to *keep the scalp loose*.

Scalp massage also promotes feelings of relaxation and well-being. He suggests that you massage your scalp

— Whenever you wash your hair, and

— When your scalp feels tight, such as when you're anxious or feel under stress.

You can also massage your scalp prior to shampooing your hair.

Preparation.

If your scalp is dry and/or tight, you can use a little warm olive oil to lubricate your fingertips. (Don't worry about oily hair; shampoo it afterwards.) If you have an oily scalp, a mixture of equal parts of witch hazel and mineral water is more suitable. If you have a normal scalp, use equal parts of rosewater and mineral water, or even water with a squeeze of lemon in it. If you have dandruff, use an anti-dandruff lotion.

Do's and don'ts.

— *Don't* use your fingernails to massage. *Do* use only the pads of your fingers (your fingertips).

— *Don't* use your palms or your whole hand. (Philip Kingsley has observed that some people massage their scalp as if polishing their car!)

— *Don't* use a plastic brush or other implement. The object of massage is to exercise the *scalp*, not the hair.

— *Don't* massage your scalp if it's at all inflamed, or if the skin is broken.

— *Do* massage gently but firmly, systematically covering the entire scalp (as will be described in the next section) until it feels warm and tingly.

How to massage your scalp.
Start at the forehead, moving to the sides (above the ears) and proceeding systematically over the crown of the head to the base of the neck. This is the direction of blood flow to the heart.

(1) Arch your hands like a tent, and place your fingertips firmly on your scalp, without exerting unnecessary pressure. Only the pads of the fingers should press against the scalp; not the fingernails.

(2) Pull the fingers together then push them apart, in a kneading motion, without lifting them or moving them through the hair.

(3) When you have massaged one area for about a minute, move to the next until your entire scalp and upper neck have been massaged.

The 'laid back' massage.
Cosmetics expert Adrien Arpel has observed that once you have mastered the rudiments of scalp massage, you don't have to do it in one position only. She has massaged her own scalp while lying on her back (supine) with her head hanging over the edge of a bed.

Philip Kingsley suggests lying on an inclined surface. I like this better because the spine is supported and there is less chance of injury. The slant board (see Chapter 6) is ideal for a lying-down massage.

Caution.
If you have high blood-pressure, a heart or breathing disorder, or weak eye capillaries, do *check with your doctor* before attempting scalp massage in this position.

Here's how the 'laid-back' massage is done:

(1) Place within easy reach a saucer or small bowl with the lubricating agent of your choice (see 'Preparation' above).

(2) Lie supine on an inclined surface, with your head lower than your feet. You may rest your head on a small pillow protected with a towel, if you wish.

(3) Dip your fingers in your container of liquid and begin your massage, as described in the previous section, starting at the forehead.

(4) Moisten your fingers before proceeding to a new area, moving backward across the head.

(5) Now turn over onto your abdomen (prone position), still with your head lower than your feet. Continue the massage from where you left off — at the crown of your head — working toward the base of your skull, the neck and the back of the ears.

(6) Using only one hand, massage one side of the neck; massage the other side with the other hand.

(7) Using both hands, finish your massage by massaging your shoulders and across the upper back.

The entire massage should last about 8 minutes and should leave you feeling wonderful.

Shampoo and shampooing
It's a fallacy that frequent shampooing is bad for hair. In fact, it may help to slow down certain types of hair loss by keeping the scalp clear of accumulated hormonal products.

Twice a week is certainly not too often to shampoo, and if your hair tends to be oily, three times weekly is not overdoing it. Some people wash their hair every day without any ill effects. I wash mine every other day, have done so for years and still receive many compliments and queries about my shiny hair.

Most shampoos, according to dermatologist Jonathan Zizmor, are essentially alkaline. If they weren't, they wouldn't be capable of dissolving grease, oil or dirt. Therefore, the very concept of an acidic or non-alkaline shampoo, is illogical. He adds that alkaline shampoos won't hurt hair since their harshness is not extreme, and can be corrected with a conditioner or cream rinse. These will close the imbrications on the cuticle of the hair shaft (see Chapter 1), which are opened by alkaline substances. Hair shines and is manageable when these imbrications are closed to form a smooth, even surface.

When it comes to the importance of pH in shampoo, Dr Zizmor claims that this is almost negligible. The measurement pH refers to the alkalinity or acidity of a product. Neutral pH is 7. Anything lower, down to 1, is progressively acidic. Anything higher, up to 14, is progressively alkaline. If you're concerned about restoring hair to a normal pH after a shampoo, you can use a conditioner, as mentioned earlier, or an acidic hair rinse (see the following section on 'Post shampoo rinse').

Perhaps more important than your choice of shampoo is your shampooing technique. Massage the scalp firmly yet gently, along the lines described in the previous section on scalp massage. Take your time, and be careful not to tug at the hair.

Hair care experts stress the need for thorough rinsing. A good, simple rule to follow is: shampoo, rinse, then rinse well again.

Conditioning and conditioners
The terms 'conditioner' and 'cream rinse' refer to approximately the same type of preparation, the latter being in liquid form.

Since all conditioners and cream rinse products are essentially mildly acidic (just as all shampoos are essentially alkaline), the concept of non-alkalinity after shampooing *is* meaningful, according to Dr Zizmor. Conditioners close imbrications on the hair cuticle opened by shampoo, and this not only protects the inner hair structure, but also imparts lustre to the surface of the hair.

In addition to closing the imbrications, nearly all conditioners seal in moisture and give body to the hair, making it easy to manage with brush or comb. This is because they usually contain some form of protein — for example, balsam. Because of their coating action, protein conditioners are especially useful in caring for fine and/or limp hair that lacks fullness. They are also good for thick, dry hair that tends to be electric following a shampoo. Other ways in which conditioners may prove helpful are for controlling split ends and post-shampoo tangles.

No conditioner or cream rinse will work wonders after a single application. To be noticeably effective it must be used regularly. Whether or not to condition your hair after each shampoo, or only once a week, depends on individual convenience and on the condition of your hair.

After shampooing your hair, apply the conditioner only to the really dry parts, omitting the areas close to the scalp. Follow instructions on product labels as to how long to leave the conditioner on your hair before rinsing it off.

For a home-made conditioner, Dr Zizmor suggests mixing three tablespoons of either apple cider vinegar or lemon juice in a glass of cool water and carefully combing the solution through wet, freshly-shampooed hair. Finish with a cool water rinse for shimmering hair.

The idea of a conditioner and shampoo combined into a single product is undoubtedly appealing to today's busy men and women: it's convenient and it promises to save time. Unfortunately, the conditioning and detergent effects of such a product counteract each other. For most individuals, then, using a separate shampoo and conditioner is a wiser practice.

Post shampoo rinse

If you're concerned about your scalp's natural pH, treat your hair to an apple cider vinegar rinse after shampooing. Mix together 15ml (1 tablespoon) apple cider vinegar and 250ml (1 cup) cool water. Pour the mixture over freshly shampooed hair and rub it in gently but well. Drape a towel around your head to absorb surplus moisture before drying your hair.

Hair drying

The ideal way to dry hair is to do so gently with an absorbent towel and carefully comb and style it with a wide-toothed comb. The air will do the rest. Today's busy persons, however, won't find this method convenient, and so the electric hairdryer has become a fact of life for them. Even so blow-dryers, especially if used on high heat settings, should not be used routinely.

Any appliance that blows hot air onto hair is potentially very drying. Used habitually, it can cause hair to become dull, brittle and full of split ends. In time the cuticle and later the inner hair structure may become damaged. The consensus of experts is therefore that it's best not to blow-dry your hair routinely.

For those of you who can't avoid routine use of a blow-dryer, however, here are some points to note:

(1) Before blow-drying wet hair, towel dry and comb it carefully.
(2) Use a blow-dryer with a low wattage, or use the low heat setting on a higher-watt model.
(3) Consider protecting your hair with one of the protein-based products now available to coat the hair and protect it from the intense heat of the blow-dryer.
(4) Start drying first the back of the head, with the hair nearest the scalp. Do the middle sections next, styling the ends last.
(5) Hold the dryer no closer than 6 to 12 inches (15 to 30 centimetres) away from the hair and scalp. Diffuse rather than concentrate the heat on any one area at a time. Use slower and cooler air-flow settings, and *never overdry* the hair. Overdrying can cause hair to weaken and fall abnormally.

Hair brushing and combing

Do not brush or comb wet hair. When hair is wet, it loses its tensile strength. At this time, it can be stretched to almost twice its usual length. Under this kind of strain, it will break easily. It is therefore wiser to comb the hair when it is dry, or almost dry. Never brush wet hair.

Avoid using plastic or metal combs, which tend to weaken the hair and damage the scalp. The best type of comb to buy, according to Philip Kingsley, is saw-cut. Each individual tooth is cut into the comb, leaving no rough or sharp edges. Saw-cut combs can be made of plastic, but vulcanite (hard rubber) ones are best.

A good quality, natural, tapered bristle brush (often made from boar's hairs) is kindest to your hair. Brushes with ball-tipped, synthetic bristles — which have now become popular — are also gentle to the scalp.

Cleaning combs and brushes.
Dissolve a tablespoon of soda in a basin of hot water. You may add a little antiseptic. Soak combs and brushes in this solution for about five minutes, then swirl them around, one at a time, until they are clean. Finally, rinse them under warm running water and place them on a clean surface to dry.

Styling options
For a well-defined, spiky hairstyle that needs plenty of hold, use a fluffy mousse. If you have thin hair, however, using a mousse may cause it to look greasy and thinner.

For a sleek, wet look, use a gel or glaze. Use a setting lotion for control and body when setting your hair with rollers.

Waving and straightening
Inherited hair genes determine whether hair is naturally straight or wavy. In order to alter the contour of the hair with which you were born, you have to resort to chemical or mechanical aids.

A single hair maintains its form — straight or wavy — by a sulfhydryl (SH) bond or linkage, which is present in specific chemical and physical proportions. It is this bond that gives hair its tensile strength. If you want to change your hair's contour, or shape, this SH bond must first be broken. The easiest way to do this is by means of chemicals, as in the waving process. Since this process tends to be repeated, the chances of hair damage increases unless extreme caution is exercised. One doctor has remarked that a choice may eventually have to be made: permanent wave or permanent hair.

With reference to a strand of hair, waving and straightening are the same thing. In either case, the hair undergoes the same three stages: softening, rearrangement of the softened hair into a new position, and chemically halting the reaction period with a special neutralizer to maintain new alignments.

Perming

Dr Zizmor advises that for your first 'permanent', you should go
to a professional hairdresser. Once you see how the procedure is
done correctly, you'll be able to do it yourself at home. With
chemical waving, you get curls that last — to some extent — until
the affected hair is cut off. The stronger the hair shaft, the better
it can accept and hold the curl. It is the cortex, not the cuticle, that
holds the wave. There is less cortex on a shaft of fine hair than on
a similar shaft of thicker hair.

Home hair permanents have the potential for generating a
variety of hair problems. These include split ends, brittle hair, and
abnormal hair loss. Fortunately, the split ends can be helped with
conditioners and cured by a haircut. If the hair follicles are
healthy, they will still be able to grow new hair to replace that
which was broken. The best preventative against these and other
problems is to follow package directions carefully. If your hair has
been recently and/or regularly bleached, reconsider before
subjecting it to permanent waving. Such hair is more liable to
damage from waving chemicals than hair not so treated.

Hair should be well cut and freshly shampooed before being
permanently waved.

Straightening

Some chemicals used in hair straightening can be caustic. Used
improperly, they can cause scalp irritations and burns. Dr Nelson
Lee Novick, author of *Skin Care for Teens*, does not recommend
steam irons for straightening hair. There is a decided risk of heat
damage to the hair and accidental burning of the scalp or skin with
this method.

Setting

The heat generated by electric hair-setting rollers breaks the
weaker hydrogen bonds in hair, thus temporarily facilitating hair
styling. Overuse of these rollers, however, can be very damaging.
It can result in dry, brittle hair, particularly if the hair is bleached
or tinted. Generally, hot-mist (steam-heated) rollers are better
than straight electric rollers because the mist replenishes some of
the moisture lost in the heating process.

Electric rollers are possibly better than overnight rollers, which may pull on the hair; but their daily use is *not* recommended. Use rollers only on thoroughly dry hair, and use end papers to prevent damaged ends.

Electric curling irons also work by weakening hydrogen bonds in hair. Since these tend to be hotter than electric rollers, however, *extreme care* should be exercised when using them. Excessive use of curling irons can result in scalp burns and in dry, brittle or burnt hair.

Bleaching and colouring

Hair care experts suggest a visit to a beauty salon as the safest and best way to learn how to part the hair and apply a bleaching agent. Professional hair bleaching has been perfected because of hydrogen peroxide which, observes Dr Zizmor, is relatively safe and cheap, and critical to the effectiveness of colouring dyes. Hydrogen peroxide opens the imbrications of the hair cuticle just enough to allow it to reach the hair shaft, without causing significant damage. Once inside, it chemically changes the melanin colouring proteins of the hair by means of oxidation.

Experts *do not* recommend repeated bleaching of the hair. They say it can damage the cuticle over time, and make the hair fragile and strawlike.

Henna

From the most ancient times, the leaves of the henna plant have been used in eastern countries to dye the hair and stain the nails. Since 1890 it has been widely used in Europe for tinting the hair, usually in the form of a shampoo. A variety of shades are available, the result of mixing the henna with other plants, for example, indigo.

Natural henna is a harmless, non-irritating, permanent dye. It's mixed in a bowl and applied to the hair, either as a rinse or a paste. It comes in a variety of shades, all of which fall into the red-to-auburn part of the spectrum. Depending on how long it's left on, it produces varying degrees of reddish highlights to the hair. It has the advantage over some other colouring agents in that it contains no artificial ingredients whatsoever. If you want to avoid the potentially harsh side-effects of certain dyes and bleaches, henna may be your answer. Henna, moreover, does not cause the imbrications of the hair cuticle to open, but rather to stay tightly closed. It does not penetrate the hair shaft. It therefore helps protect the hair and make it glossier. Periodic applications deposit additional protective coatings, thus increasing the diameter of each hair strand, and therefore hair volume.

Henna is not without some limitations, however. Darker shades are unsuitable for light blond hair or hair that's more than 20 per cent grey. An alternative for such hair is to treat it first with a neutral or strawberry henna. Mixtures of any other shade can then be applied.

Occasional build-up problems may also occur, but all in all, henna works very well.

For special effects, try other herbs in the form of a rinse after your henna treatment. Red Zinger tea will enrich red tones; camomile will lighten the tone, and beet juice will intensify reds.

Natural hennas, although adding no colour, will make thin or fine hair appear thicker.

Care for tinted hair:
— Shampoo less frequently; lather once only.
— Use a conditioner after shampooing.
— Avoid exposure to the sun.
— Avoid swimming in chlorinated water unless you use a hair conditioner or wear a bathing cap.

Split ends
A split end, or mid-shaft split, occurs when the hair cuticle is damaged and the fibres of the cortex unravel. Split ends are also known as 'the frizzies'.

One of the main causes of split ends is over-treatment with bleaches and chemical dyes; but all chemical treatments have the potential to damage the hair's protective cuticle. Ragged or ruined cuticles not only lead to split ends, but also produce dull, unmanageable hair. Another major cause of split ends is overmanipulation of the hair: too much brushing, too much teasing, heavy brushes with sharp bristles and careless use of brush rollers.

Overheating is another factor contributing to split ends: overuse of electric rollers, curling irons, hot-oil treatments and blowdryers can scorch the cuticle. Once the cuticle is weakened, the shaft will eventually split. One other cause of the frizzies is humidity. On a rainy day, for instance, hair will suck up water from the air and swell. Split ends will then be more noticeable.

Preventing split ends
If you're troubled with split ends, you may need to reduce the number of times you wash your hair. You will also need to avoid undue exposure to the sun. The sun's ultraviolet (UV) rays can damage the cuticle. If you swim in a chlorine-treated pool and then follow it with a sauna, the combination of chlorine and dehydration from the heat will damage even normally healthy hair.

Conditioners will temporarily help in treating split ends. The only real cure, however, is to cut the split ends off.

Hair in pregnancy
There are two major causes of hair problems during and immediately following pregnancy: changes in the normal balance of hormones, and pregnancy-related stress.

During pregnancy, hair tends to be dryer than usual. Due to hormonal changes, however, scalp hair is more abundant. Hair care at this time should be kept simple. Hair should be treated as if it were dry, because it usually is. If you need to wash it every day, do so, but don't counteract the effects of washing with harsh blowdrying. Use a shampoo and conditioner made for dry hair.

Be sure that your diet is adequate. You may want to look again at Chapter 3.

After pregnancy
Two or three months after the baby is born, a woman can expect hair loss, which can sometimes be dramatic and frightening. Often at some point between the second and seventh months postpartum, hair that didn't fall out during pregnancy combines with

hair that is regularly shed. The cause is a re-adjustment of hormonal balance, which can also result in dandruff and greasy hair. This sudden, increased hair fall is known as *post-partum alopecia* (pronounced 'al-o-pee-she-ah'), and is aggravated by stress. In most cases, however, the hair returns to normal between the second and eighth month after delivery.

To treat post-partum alopecia, the first thing to do is to learn to *calm down*. You may want to review Chapter 6, but please *check with your doctor* before practising the physical exercises prescribed. Also consult your doctor to rule out other possible causes of abnormal hair fall.

Because hair will be greasier than usual after delivery, use a very mild shampoo, and wash your hair daily if you can.

Time of Month

Premenstrually a woman's hair tends to be at its worst. If it's usually greasy, it will be greasier; if dandruff is generally a problem, it will be more so at this time of month. Hair fall may be more pronounced.

The key to treatment is to simplify hair care. If your hair is dryer, use a shampoo and conditioner made for dry hair. If it is greasier, use a very mild shampoo and wash your hair daily if you can.

For hints on how to cope with dandruff, read the following section entitled 'Hair's friends and foes'.

Don't worry unnecessarily about increased hair fall. Learn to relax (see Chapter 6). Get adequate exercise, out of doors if possible, and enough sleep. Be conscientious about eating a wholesome diet, and drink plenty of water (see Chapter 3).

For further information on overcoming menstrual and related problems, do read my book entitled *Pain-free Periods* (see Bibliography).

Hair's friends and foes

Food. Highly processed foods of all kinds, habitually consumed, are bad for hair. They provide only 'empty calories' which result in weak, dull hair. Unprocessed foods, by contrast, are kind to the whole body and therefore to the hair. They furnish essential nutrients which build health. This health is reflected in luxuriant hair which enhances your appeal and self-confidence.

Beverages. Coffee, tea, cocoa and cola drinks contain compounds called *xanthines.* These substances include caffeine, theophylline and theobromine, which are powerful stimulants. They act on the nervous, respiratory (breathing), and cardiovascular (heart and blood vessels) systems. They increase the excretion of water and important nutrients from the body. They can be highly irritating to persons sensitive to them.

Healthful alternatives to tea, coffee, cocoa and cola drinks include: water, unsweetened fruit juices, mineral water, milk and herbal teas.

Alcohol is a mixed blessing. It does give diameter to blood vessels and so facilitates blood flow to the tissues. It is, however, antagonistic to several minerals and vitamins that are essential to healthy hair. If you want to keep hair on your head, therefore, and you want to keep it healthy and attractive, do limit your alcohol intake to an occasional drink or two.

Contraceptive pills. These are potential enemies of your hair. Their undesirability lies essentially in the fact that they act against nutrients crucial to hair health, such as the B-complex vitamins and zinc.

Stress. Here's another agent that's inimical to hair. It may, in fact, be your hair's worst enemy. Following are some ill effects stress produces:

— It causes excessive sweating which, combined with dust and other airborne pollutants, clogs the pores of the scalp.

— It increases the tension of muscles, which then compress underlying blood vessels and restrict blood circulation to tissue supporting the hair.

— It increases secretion of the sebaceous (oil-producing) glands, which contributes to dandruff formation.

Philip Kingsley has stated that stress is unquestionably the single most dangerous circumstance a career woman encounters. It is highly injurious not only to the health of her hair, but also to the rest of her body. (This applies to men as well.)

For more information on stress, please refer to Chapter 6.

Sun. Sun is as bad for hair as it is for skin. It degrades the hair shaft, making it weak and dull looking. Do wear a hat or scarf whenever practicable, or sit in a shaded area.

Lack of exercise. Every single cell of the body depends on an adequate blood supply for health and renewal. When the blood has to travel 'uphill' as it does to reach cells making up the scalp, it has to contend with the forces of gravity. Not infrequently, it reaches its destination diminished and sometimes impoverished. The hair's manufacturing plant (the hair bulb and papillae), situated beneath the scalp, does not receive all the raw materials it needs to make healthy hair and hair production suffers as a result.

Regular exercise beneficially stimulates the circulatory and other intimately related systems: the respiratory, nervous, endocrine and lymphatic. It encourages a healthful blood supply to vital structures, nourishing them adequately and helping them regenerate and repair themselves. Exercise, moreover, is an excellent tension reliever — one of the best available antidotes against stress.

In addition to aerobic exercise such as brisk walking, running, bicycling, swimming or tennis, I suggest regular practice of a semi-inverted posture such as *The Shoulderstand*, described and illustrated in Chapter 7, or lying on a *Slant Board* (see Chapter 6), unless of course you have some condition that forbids it.

At the very least, practise the *Legs Up* exercise daily (described in Chapter 6), combining it with slow, rhythmical breathing to promote deep relaxation of the whole body.

You would also benefit from regularly practising shoulder and neck warm-ups (see Chapter 7) every day to discourage tension build up as this quickly spreads to the face, scalp and other parts of the body. Tension, it bears repeating, effectively reduces the free flow of blood to tissues thus diminishing the nutrition these structures receive.

Traction. Anything that increases scalp tension is injurious to the hair. Tight curlers, perms, braids and pony-tails and tugging at the hair while shampooing or styling it are all forms of mechanical stress which contribute to traction baldness.

Dandruff. Also known as seborrhoea, this has already been dealt with in Chapter 5. In treating this condition, the first step to take is to determine the cause or causes. For this, you may need to consult your doctor who may then refer you to a dermatologist.

Meanwhile, here are several things you can do to help control the disorder:

— Keep your hair and scalp scrupulously clean. Use a natural anti-dandruff shampoo (available in health food stores), provided this is compatible with treatment prescribed by your doctor. Also, keep combs and brushes immaculate.

— Avoid overprocessed foods. Stick to a wholesome diet.

— Exercise regularly. This will, among many other benefits, facilitate the elimination of wastes from your body.

— Incorporate relaxation techniques into your daily schedule to help you cope effectively with stress.

For more in-depth information on hair and all aspects of hair care, you may wish to read my book entitled *The Secrets of Stopping Hair Loss* (see Bibliography).

9. SKIN DEEP AND MORE

Skin has become an important object of attention in the health care movement. We've at last acknowledged that skin is not merely a means of protection for vital structures but itself a major one. It is in fact our largest organ, representing about 15 per cent of our body weight.

Although the skin is plainly visible, looking after it is not an external affair only but also an internal matter. Thoughtful professionals therefore approach skin care both from within and without.

Like all other body tissues, skin needs nourishment from the inside to be healthy and to repair itself when damaged. Chapter 3 deals at some length with nutrients which are of particular importance to the skin, and gives information about foods richest in these substances.

EFAs
Crucial to optimum skin health and attractiveness, EFAs (essential fatty acids) are discussed in depth in Chapter 2.

EFAs are a necessary component of the oils that lubricate the skin and keep it resilient. They play a vital role in the structure of each of the billions of cells that make up our skin. They influence the passage of solutes through the cell wall (permeability). They are also very important for the maintenance of membrane fluidity. According to Judy Graham, author of *Evening Primrose Oil* (see Bibliography), how fluid and flexible cell membranes are depends on how many EFAs they contain. In addition, EFAs are imperative for keeping the skin waterproof.

With these EFA functions in mind, your choice of moisturizing skin cream or lotion will not be difficult. Select a product that will help reduce transepidermal (literally 'across the epidermis') water loss; a product that serves a natural moisturizing function.

EFA trials and studies

Many recent studies and trials have been conducted, using evening primrose oil (EPO) to treat various skin conditions. From the results of this research, it is apparent that this amazing oil offers substantial hope for restoring and maintaining the integrity of the skin.

It is important to realize that not all EPOs are created equal. Unless their GLA content is adequate, they are worthless. The choice of a GLA source seems clear: EPO contains GLA; GLA can by-pass certain blockages occurring during EFA metabolism. It is the factor that offers protection against certain eczemas and other skin disorders.

Best skin care products

Cosmetic skin creams and lotions usually have an oil base. Manufacturers of most preparations on the market use oils that won't spoil. These products give a certain protection to the skin against the drying effects of sun, wind and rain. They coat the skin but don't actively support skin nutrition and health. This is because they lack EFAs.

The best skin care products always contain EFAs, which are readily absorbable. Non-organic grease (for example, petroleum jelly) is not absorbed at all.

Several skin care preparations containing EFAs are available in Europe, where knowledge of skin health is more advanced than in certain other parts of the world. Such products are now increasingly obtainable in North America, and can usually be found in health food stores.

The first ingredient for which to look when choosing skin care products is evening primrose oil (EPO). EPO is easily absorbable, especially when applied to the abdomen and inner surface of the arms. Its external application complements the internal use of the oil as an excellent source of GLA which is very well received by the body.

Skin permeability

The skin's capability of allowing the passage of fluids or substances is referred to as its *permeability*. If the epidermis is a barrier to substances entering the body, how can anything penetrate the skin?

The probable route is by way of the follicles and sebaceous glands. You may find it convenient to think of the follicles as minute tunnels in the skin through which substances can enter, and thence via the sebaceous ducts to the deeper tissues. It is noteworthy that fat-miscible and fat-soluble substances have the greatest potential to penetrate skin.

Worthy of note, too, is that persons suffering from atopic eczema (see Chapter 5) may develop asthma when certain types of protein, such as egg white, are applied to their skin. This is only one example of the fact that, although skin acts as a barrier to some agents, others can penetrate it and be absorbed by it.

More on skin care products

Apart from the EPO in the skin care products you purchase, you should also look for certain other ingredients that will protect, nourish, repair and heal the skin day or night, winter or summer. The products you buy should have the capability of maintaining the skin's moisture balance and so help prevent undue water loss across this protective barrier. When skin is dry, its elasticity diminishes and premature ageing occurs.

The skin care products you select should counteract the effects of sun and wind and daily wear and tear, keeping it smooth, supple and wonderful to touch.

Another important consideration in choosing the skin care products you will be using habitually is this: they should have been tested *on humans* and found non-irritating.

Worthy of note are products containing any of the following ingredients: aloe vera, bee pollen, calendula, chamomile, jojoba oil, and various minerals and vitamins.

When shopping for deep-pore cleansing scrubs, look for those with almond meal, apricot seeds, corn meal, oatmeal, rye flour, or sea salt, and herbs with cleansing and healing abilities.

In choosing cleansers, ingredients to look for include camphor, eucalyptus, menthol and witch hazel.

Don't forget to take advantage of NaPCA to improve the moisturization of your skin, and consequently its look and feel. NaPCa (sodium pyrrolidone carboxylate) is a non-oily, very effective humectant that is now available in a handy spray bottle. Spray it over your body after bathing, or on your face before applying makeup.

Checking out the products

In a capsule, here are the criteria by which to judge the creams and lotions you will be using habitually on your skin. The products you choose and use should contain:

— a clinically well tested brand of EPO;

— vitamin A, 'the skin vitamin', which enhances the conversion of GLA to PGE1;

— vitamin E, to shield the skin from disturbing environmental influences, for example sunlight;

— UVA and UVB filters, to protect skin from the sun's damaging rays;

— agents to soothe, condition and heal the skin.

Your skin care products should also have a mild, pleasing fragrance, acceptable to you and other family members and associates. Do *avoid* products with perfumes which, in combination with the sun, may produce an allergic reaction.

— Choose a non-occlusive product, that is, one that does not obstruct the skin's tiny openings (e.g. pores).

— Select a non-greasy product that slips obligingly into the skin so that you're conscious of its effect rather than its presence.

— Use a product that will impart a sleek, youthful appearance to the skin, and which will be a decided pleasure to use at any time.

Sun and skin

Countless magazine and television advertisements extol the virtues of sun-tanned skin. They are designed to persuade us that a sun-bronzed body is a symbol of health and success, and many persons are so swayed. They take every opportunity to bask in the sun or otherwise expose themselves to it, despite repeated warnings that such exposure can, and will, eventually harm their skin — indeed their whole body.

Sun is the number one cause of premature ageing of the skin. The old, tired, leather-like, dehydrated skin that's a consequence of over-exposure to the sun's rays is dubbed by the nursing profession 'the Miami Beach syndrome'. It's the dubious reward of many sunny hours spent in the garden, on the beach or on ship's deck.

It is true that the sun does some good. It converts substances in the skin into vitamin D. This vitamin is essential for a sound bony framework and for the absorption of nutrients such as calcium. The sun also helps convert carotene into vitamin A (see Chapter 3), which is of the utmost importance to the health of skin, hair and nails. Moreover, because the sun's ultraviolet rays destroy bacteria, they can be of value in clearing up some skin conditions such as acne and psoriasis.

When the sun shines, people tend to feel better than when it's cloudy or raining. Sunshine also helps relieve some of the discomforts associated with health disorders like asthma and arthritis. But there is a negative side to all this, and the disadvantages of much exposure to sun, it seems, far outweigh the advantages.

How sun damages the skin

Sun damages the elastin fibres that give elasticity to the skin. It destroys the collagen holding together the cells that make up skin tissue and give it strength. As we age and our epidermis becomes thinner, this destructive process becomes easier. The skin dries out and hardens, sometimes leading to *solar keratosis* (horn-like skin growths caused by sun), which appears as rough, scaly patches that often precede cancer.

The sun's ultraviolet radiation also damages the DNA (deoxy-ribonucleic acid) — the genetic material, or 'blueprint', in the cells. In time, accumulated DNA damage can set the scene for the formation of cancer cells. Some authorities now go as far as stating that skin cancer is not merely linked to the sun, but is actually caused by it.

Skin cancer

Skin cancer is the most common type of cancer. In nine out of ten cases, the cancer occurs in uncovered parts of the body: the face, ears, neck and back of the hands.

According to a recent article appearing in *Newsweek* magazine, the most common dangers from sun exposure are basal- and squamous-cell carcinoma (cancer). Luckily, these are curable if detected early. The outcome of the third, rarer, type of cancer is not so fortunate. It's called *malignant melanoma* and its incidence has risen from one in every 1,500 persons in 1930 to one in every 150 at present — an alarming tenfold increase.

Evidence suggests that malignant melanoma is caused by one or more serious sunburns in childhood or adolescence, rather than by the cumulative effects of sun exposure. In all three carcinomas, the active ingredient is the sun's ultraviolet radiation.

When EFAs are a regular part of the diet, they are present in the skin and absorb sunlight for future use in vital biochemical reactions. It is worthy of note that cancer victims often lack these EFAs and are therefore more vulnerable to sunburn. Sun-caused skin cancers are also linked to deficiencies of vitamin A and vitamin B_6.

More on sun damage

The sun's ultraviolet (UV) rays penetrate the skin's layers very well indeed. They can, in fact, reach the dermis, the important structural part of the skin. It is the dermis that gives skin its shape, strength and elasticity. UV light changes the physical character-istics of the dermis from thick, strong, resilient tissue to a thin, weak, inelastic one. The skin begins to wrinkle and sag, and unfortunately does so more markedly in fair-skinned people who don't make and disperse enough pigment to block UV light from their dermis (see Bibliography: Goodman).

Other signs of early skin ageing through sun damage are dark patches known as 'age spots' and wrinkles around the eyes, on the upper lip and on the neck and hands.

You can become sunburned without realizing it, as on a cloudy day or while swimming. You can suffer a sunburn even when your skin doesn't turn red while you're in the sun. In fact, your skin doesn't reach maximum redness until about eight hours after you have been in the sun. It's not only fair-skinned blondes and freckled redheads who suffer sunburn. Dark-skinned people are also vulnerable.

Solar radiation

The UV (ultraviolet) component of sunlight induces normal and abnormal changes in the skin. UV radiation is subdivided into UVA, UVB and UVC.

UVA rays, sometimes called tanning rays, are of long wave length (320 to 400 nanometres). It penetrates well into the dermis, causing both immediate and delayed tanning (melanogenesis). It can also evoke a weak sunburn reaction. UVA radiation can also produce a photosensitivity reaction to certain drugs, cosmetics and other substances (see the next section).

UVB rays, or mid-range UV (290 to 320 nanometres) are responsible for sunburn and delayed tanning. The energy from UVB radiation has also been implicated in causing wrinkling and skin cancer (through its effect on the DNA of the epidermis).

Window glass allows UVA rays to pass through, while filtering out UVB radiation.

The shortest wave length in the UV spectrum is UVC (200 to 290 nanometres). It is sometimes referred to as germicidal (germ-killing) radiation. Because UVC is effectively screened by the ozone layer in the atmosphere, it does not reach the earth's surface.

UVC radiation is also emitted by artificial sources such as germicidal lamps, welding arcs and high- and low-pressure mercury arc lamps, and is considered potentially carcinogenic (cancer-producing). Individuals exposed to UVC radiation from artificial sources may experience a mild reddening of the skin (erythema).

Photosensitivity and phototoxicity

The prefix of these two words ('photo') comes from the Greek word *photos* which means 'light'.

Photosensitivity, then, literally means 'sensitivity to light' and is the same as *photoallergy*. It is a response that occurs when light rays interact with certain chemicals, such as the phenothiazines, sulfonamides, some sunscreen agents, bleaches and anti-histamines.

Phototoxicity pertains to the harmful reaction produced by light energy, particularly by the sun on the skin. A sunburn is one example of phototoxicity.

Sun does not mix well with certain substances. In some individuals, such an unhappy combination can produce burns, blotches or rashes (photosensitivity). Other agents produce an adverse reaction in everyone (phototoxic substances). One common phototoxic agent is essence of lime, an ingredient in some lime-scented colognes and after-shave lotions. Another is oil of bergamot, used in some perfumes.

Photosensitivity may also occur in some women who use birth control pills. Unsightly dark brown patches may appear on the cheeks and upper lip. The marks usually disappear, though, when the contraceptive pills are discontinued.

Some antibiotics can cause photosensitivity. Tetracycline, commonly used to treat acne, is one of them, although it doesn't often produce this reaction. The antibiotic Declomycin, on the other hand, has a photosensitizing effect on 99 per cent of persons using it.

Antifungal pills used to treat athlete's foot, some artificial sweeteners such as saccharin and cyclamates (common in diet foods and soft drinks) and the halogenated salicylamides, an ingredient in deodorant soaps, are other common photosensitizers. A combination of sun exposure and using tranquillizers or diuretics ('water pills') can also occasionally lead to a bad skin burn. The ingredients in some cosmetics and perfumes can sometimes cause adverse reactions.

The juice from certain fruits and vegetables (e.g., celery, figs, limes, parsley, parsnips) and some flowers (e.g., chrysanthemums, marigolds and morning glory) can cause sun poisoning.

If you are taking medications or using any products containing ingredients mentioned in this section, please *check with your doctor* before planning to sunbathe. In any event, you should protect yourself adequately from undue exposure to the sun at all times.

What's your skin type?

Skin types are rated from one to six, depending on the degree of sunburn experienced in the initial 35-40 minutes of unprotected exposure to sun.

Skin type category	Description
I	Always burns easily; never tans (**sensitive**)
II	Always burns easily; tans minimally (**sensitive**)
III	Burns moderately; tans gradually and evenly (**normal**)
IV	Burns minimally; always tans well (**normal**)
V	Rarely burns; tans deeply (**insensitive**)
VI	Never burns; deeply pigmented (**insensitive**)

Choosing a sunscreen

Having determined your skin type, you can now intelligently select the product best suited to your complexion and which will produce the desired effect. Sunscreen products are rated according to SPF, or sun protection factor, currently numbering between 2 and 30, depending on their protective value.

SPF is a standard established by the US Federal Drug

Authority indicating the length of time a sunscreen keeps the skin from burning. For example, a cream or lotion with an SPF of 2, properly applied, allows users to stay in the sun twice as long as they could without protection.

The Skin Cancer Foundation and many skin specialists recommend the use of a sunblocking agent with an SPF of at least 15 for the face, and regular use of moisturizers containing sunscreens. The sun's rays, after all, reach most of us all year long.

SPF Number	Effects
2	Gives minimal protection only, but does permit sun-tanning. *Suitable* for persons with skin type VI, but best used after previous exposure to sun. *Unsuitable* for light-complexioned adults and small children.
4	Moderate sunscreen, permitting some tanning. *Suitable* for persons with skin no lighter than type V.
6	Moderate sun protection, permitting limited, gradual tanning. *Suitable* for individuals with skin type IV.
8	'Maximal sunscreen' which, although affording extra protection, eventually permits some tanning. *Suitable* for persons with skin type III.
15	'Ultra' sun protection. Offers the most protection from sun burning. Tanning may occur very slowly. *Especially suitable* for blondes, red-heads and fair-skinned individuals.

SPF Number	Effects
23–25	Intended to be a complete sun block, protecting from both UVA and UVB rays. Having the potential as the most effective preventive against skin cancer.
30	Use of a sunscreen with SPF 30 or more is unnecessary and may be detrimental, because the additional chemicals in these preparations decrease moisturization and are therefore not good for the skin.

Please note that European SPF numbers are lower than those cited in this section, which appear on North American products. A European number 5, for example, would be the equivalent of an American number 10.

When shopping for a sunscreen, here are tips to help you select one that's right for you. Effective sunscreens should be:

— nontoxic,

— nondiscolouring,

— nonirritating and nonsensitizing (i.e., innocuous),

— cosmetically acceptable.

Sunscreen products are available in creams (oily or vanishing), lotions (clear or milky) and gels. Consider these factors before making your choice:

— Skin type. For example, if you have a fair complexion and blue, green or grey eyes; if you burn easily and tan poorly, you should buy a sunscreen with an SPF of at least 10.

— Type of activity. If you engage in water sports, such as swimming or windsurfing, or sweat profusely (after exercising, for example), select a product with good substantivity (that is, one that resists removal when subjected to moisture).

— If you snow-ski or mountain climb, you would benefit from a sunscreen with a higher SPF than you usually use, because of the added effects of UV radiation at higher altitude, and the reflective properties of snow.

— The nose and lips are particularly sensitive to UV radiation, so maximum protection of these areas is required. Physical sunscreens such as zinc oxide may be used on these vulnerable areas, but these agents are not cosmetically acceptable to most people. Gel-based products for the lips may be preferable. An opaque lipstick may be used after applying sunscreen.

— If you have dry skin, you may benefit from a sunscreen with a cream or lotion base. If your skin is oily (especially if it is prone to acne), you would do better with an alcohol solution or gel. Sunscreens with an alcohol base should *not* however, be used on eczematous or inflamed skin.

— If you exhibit a photosensitivity reaction or have a condition that is exacerbated by exposure to sunlight (for example, lupus), products with PABA or PABA esters are not suitable for you. This is because such products do not absorb the UVA radiation that is responsible for photosensitivity reactions.

Protection from the sun

The only natural defence of significance which unprotected skin has against UV radiation is provided by melanin in the epidermis. Melanin is the pigment that gives colour to skin and hair. When skin is exposed to sunlight, special melanin-forming cells called melanocytes release granules of protective pigment (melanin), which absorb and scatter subsequent doses of UV. The longer the exposure, the greater this dispersion of melanin.

The sun's tanning rays also trigger an increase in the melanocytes and in the production of new granules. All these factors combined lead to an increasingly darker tan. But the process is not foolproof.

Long-term exposure to sunlight causes substantial cumulative damage to the skin. The major changes are in pigment and skin texture. They are collectively known as *photoageing*. The chief manifestations are atrophy, dryness, splotchy hypo- or hyperpigmentation (often seen on sun-exposed areas of middle-aged or older persons), telangiectasia (dilation of capillaries) and, of course, wrinkling. In addition, solar elastosis can occur. This refers to the loss of normal elastic and connective tissue in the upper dermis. Bruising easily is one consequence of this.

Fair-skinned individuals are understandably more susceptible to these skin changes; but pigmented skin resists photoageing only partially. However, the most serious long-term effect of sunlight on skin, as mentioned earlier, is skin cancer.

Here is something else to think about. A study carried out at the University of Sydney in Australia revealed that the human immune system could be noticeably depressed for up to two weeks following exposure to UVA rays.

Researcher Vicki O'Brien (see Bibliography) advises that if you want healthy skin you should stop tanning yourself. This advice notwithstanding, large numbers of persons will continue to seek and avail themselves of opportunities to acquire a deep sun tan which, they tell themselves, is an unquestionable mark of superb health and a symbol of prosperity.

If you are one of these persons — and even if you are not — the following tips will alert you to precautions you should be taking as you prepare to bare your body to the sun's seductive rays. Conscientiously applied, the hints to follow will help you maintain the best possible skin condition.

— Wear a wide-brimmed hat or carry a parasol, whenever practicable, if you're going to spend much time in the sun. Wear long trousers and long-sleeved garments.

— Apply a sunscreen suitable for your skin. Make sure it isn't rubbed or washed off during exposure to the sun. To ensure the very best skin protection, use a product with an SPF (sun protection factor) number of 8 or more.

Apply your sunscreen at least 30 minutes before you go out into the sunshine. Pay special attention to the ears, face, back and sides of the neck, the upper chest and back, and the back of the hands and forearms. Reapply the sunscreen after swimming or sweating profusely.

— The sun's damaging UV rays can penetrate clothing. Do limit the time spent in the sun, even when you're fully clothed.

— Avoid sunning yourself during the four hours around noon (between ten in the morning and two in the afternoon). During this time, the sun is more intense than earlier or later.

— When preparing for a ski trip, use a sunscreen with an SPF number of 15, and be especially careful to give protection to your lips.

— Consider using a makeup base that contains a sunscreen. Even when you're not sunbathing, and even on cloudy days and in the winter, your face is exposed to the sun's rays. Over the years, this exposure can be substantial.

— Don't ever use deodorant soaps on your face, or on any other part of your body that will be exposed to the sun. These soaps are photosensitizing and can cause you to burn badly.

— Wear sunglasses, not only to protect the eyes from UV radiation and keep vision more comfortable, but also to prevent squinting, which accentuates wrinkles around the eyes.

Winter skin care

Winter's icy winds combine with the low humidity of outdoor cold and indoor heat to produce dry skin and cracked lips. What happens is this: blood vessels dilate to bring a better blood flow to the skin to warm it. More moisture therefore reaches the skin surface and greater evaporation takes place.

Experts offer these tips to help you deal effectively with winter's assaults on your skin and keep it in the best possible condition.

— Use a very gentle cleanser that will not remove too much of the skin's natural oils.

— Regularly apply a cream with rich emollients to help keep the skin well moisturized and protected.

— Skin on the lips is unlike skin elsewhere on the body. Its delicate mucous membrane is easily damaged by chronic over-exposure to the elements and over-heated indoor environments. Use a lipstick rich in moisturizers and which also contains a sunscreen. It's best to wet the lips before applying any lip balm so as to lock in the moisture.

— Avoid heavy, greasy products that can damage clothing. Select and use a non-occlusive product, which doesn't plug sebaceous glands. Skin needs to breathe.

— Use a humidifier at home or in the work place to help

moisturize dry air. Alternatively, place shallow pans of water on or under radiators.

— To avoid rough, dry hands, and rigid cuticles, massage them regularly with a rich moisturizing cream and wear lined gloves outdoors.

— Generously cream feet and toenails after every wash. Wear bed socks afterwards, if appropriate.

— Take quick showers instead of prolonged baths, and use warm or cool rather than hot water to prevent dryness of the skin. Apply a moisturizer to the body within three minutes of showering.

— Avoid washing your face immediately before going outside, unless you first moisturize it adequately.

— Shower and dry yourself well after an exercise 'workout', especially after swimming in chlorinated water, which can irritate the skin.

— Avoid keeping on a damp bathing suit or swimming trunks for too long. The same applies to leotards. The combination of moisture, heat and friction from such practices may generate skin problems. Try wearing a T-shirt under your leotard.

— Drink plenty of water to keep lips and skin elsewhere on the body well hydrated and less vulnerable to chapping and cracking. Internal dehydration is a common cause of dry skin and chapped lips. People tend to drink less water in winter because they don't feel as thirsty as in warmer months. They are apt to consume more alcholic beverages and coffee, though. In addition, there are usually more colds and 'flu in winter. All these factors contribute to dehydration which takes its toll on the skin.

Indoor tanning

When health clubs, beauty parlours and tanning salons advertise indoor tanning, they endeavour to persuade prospective clients that they offer a 'safe tan'. But according to specialists, there's no such thing as a 'safe tan'.

The industry group that promotes indoor tanning is the Suntanning Association for Education (SAFE), located in Atlanta, Georgia, USA. The group readily admits that the centres offering 'safe tanning' and other 'beauty' services constitute a multi-million dollar industry.

The fact is that too much exposure to UV rays can cause premature ageing, serious eye problems such as cataracts, and cancer. In fact, the lamps used in tanning salons emit as much as ten times the UVA radiation obtained from natural sunlight, and so may be especially hazardous to skin and eyes.

Tanning booths are actually 'suntan closets' with reflective walls and vertical rows of fluorescent sunlamps. They may give you a tan, but the UV radiation they emit can also damage your skin and eyes and increase the risk of skin cancer, as mentioned above.

Until a few years ago, almost all sunlamps emitted only UVB light. People using them became tanned but they burned as well. Manufacturers then developed lamps which, they said, gave off only UVA emissions. They also told consumers that UVA rays were safer. Researchers found, however, that UVA rays were at least as damaging as UVB. In fact, UVA rays penetrate deeper into the skin than UVB rays, causing damage to collagen, blood vessels and elastic tissues. Moreover, once exposed to UVA rays, your body becomes more vulnerable to the ageing and carcinogenic effects of UVB radiation.

Tanning parlours can be set up by anyone, and tanning booth operators in many cases don't even need a licence. Some manufacturers of tanning equipment claim that their lamps emit only UVA light (which they tell consumers is safer than UVB light, but it is not). In fact, these lamps give off up to 5 per cent UVB rays. In addition, a recent study of 16 tanning salons revealed that none of the salons required the use of protective goggles, and that several didn't even supply them. In addition, some activator or accelerator creams sold by tanning services may contain *psoralens*, a chemical that makes skin more sensitive to UVA radiation.

Nevertheless, many individuals are still attracted to indoor tanning. They believe that the perceived benefits are worth the potential risks. They say that they find it therapeutic; that they feel better with a tan. They also claim that they tan indoors to develop a 'base' which, they insist, protects them from burning easily when they take a mid-winter vacation. This is a myth, however, because an indoor tan does not offer protection from the damaging effects of UV radiation, including cancer. In fact, it may add to the hazards posed by natural sunlight, since all radiation effects are cumulative.

Because of all these hazards, the American Medical Association, the American Academy of Dermatology, the US Food and Drug Administration and many dermatologists all advise against tanning, indoors or out. Of 50 patients diagnosed with skin cancer in June 1987, 70 per cent had been in a tanning parlour, and more than half were under 28 years of age.

Precautions

Regardless of risks, however, many individuals will not be able to resist the lure of the golden glow that often accompanies a tan. If you are one of these, here are some safety tips to note and apply, so as to keep damage to an absolute minimum.

— *Check with a dermatologist* first, to see if you have any pre-cancerous spots, or if your skin is too fair to be subjected to UV radiation. If you're taking medications (e.g., birth control pills, antibiotics, tranquillizers, diuretics, or medications to regulate high blood-pressure and/or diabetes) *check with your doctor or chemist* before using a tanning booth.

— Begin with short intervals, slowly building up exposure times.

— *Don't* tamper with the timer.

— Use protective goggles; simply closing your eyes or using ordinary sunglasses or cotton balls is not enough to protect your eyes. Goggles should be worn when using both UVA and UVB tanning booths.

— Avoid direct exposure to the lamps. Tanning booths should have physical barriers, such as screens or shields, to protect you from touching or falling into the lamps.

— Booths should have railings or other devices to help you keep your balance and maintain a proper distance from the heat source. Use these rails.

— Be sure that an attendant is nearby to help you in an emergency.

Note well.

You should *not* use a tanning booth (1) if you get frequent cold sores. UV radiation may worsen their appearance; (2) if you sunburn easily (usually persons with very light complexions, blond hair, and light eyes); (3) if you have dysplasic naevi, indicated by the presence of irregular moles; (4) if you have a sunburn or chronically damaged skin; (5) if your family has a history of skin cancer; (6) if you have a disorder that makes you highly photosensitive (e.g., systemic lupus erythematosus, pemphigus, or vitiligo).

Tanning at home

— *Don't* wear any cosmetics when tanning.

— *Don't* shower or take a sauna before tanning. When you towel dry yourself, you remove some natural protective body oils.

— *Do* wear goggles or other suitably protective eyewear. *Never* look at an operating sunlamp without wearing appropriate eye protection.

— *Always* follow the manufacturer's instructions regarding distance, exposure times and frequency of exposure. If there are no instructions, obtain the manufacturer's advice before you use the lamp.

— *Always* use the automatic timer to set exposure time, according to the manufacturer's recommendations. If the lamp has no timer, use some other timing device that will clearly alert you that your preset time interval has elapsed. Start the timer the instant the lamp is switched on. *Do not* tamper with the timer while you tan.

— Start your exposure schedule with a short time period; gradually increase the time for subsequent exposures. This will help build up melanin protection against skin damage.

— If you notice any immediate reddening of the skin (erythema), *stop exposure at once*. Tanning effects should not be visible for at least a few hours after exposure.

Quick-tanning products

There are a number of products that may either be ingested or applied to the body as lotions. These are generally more expensive than sunscreens or regular tanning lotions. Not infrequently, such products produce disappointing results. Some cause the palms of the hands and soles of the feet to take on an orange colour; some lotions may produce streaking of the skin. Oral products have not been proven harmless, and some dermatologists are sceptical of their protective value against the sun's most harmful rays.

Cancer alert

Although skin cancer is one of the most common cancers, the cure rate is about 90 per cent. But it is important to have it diagnosed early. If you notice any of the following, *see your doctor as soon as possible*:

— a spreading skin growth, which may be pearly, tan, brown or black in colour;

— a mole, birthmark or beauty spot that changes or takes on an odd shape;

— an open sore that doesn't heal.

Hurry to your doctor if you discover any bluish-black or dark brown, oddly shaped growths, or if the growth itches or bleeds. Malignant melanoma spreads rapidly, but it can be cured if treated early.

Treating sunburn

Sunburn is usually the result of UVB radiation, but it may also be a response to excessive UVC from artificial light sources, or to UVA in the presence of a topical photosensitizing agent (see the section on photosensitivity and phototoxicity earlier in this chapter). Although a sunburn is most commonly seen after overexposure to sun, it may also follow exposure to sunlamps or occupational light sources, such as welding arcs or photo-engraving, bactericidal or cold quartz lamps.

The simplest remedy for a mild sunburn is to apply cool tap water compresses for 20 minutes three or four times a day to the sunburned areas.

One doctor's suggested treatment for mild sunburns is to apply vinegar. Another simple sunburn reliever is to wet a towel in a solution of strong cold tea and apply it to the sunburned areas.

Dr Zizmor's recipe for a soothing and pain-relieving compress is to add two tablespoons of salt to a quart of milk, mix these together, and add some crushed ice. Dip a clean cloth into the solution and apply it to the affected parts. You might also like to check out products containing aloe vera. They are formulated to help alleviate pain and restore moisture to dehydrated skin. Some help prevent the formation of blisters and scars.

If you wish, you may apply a suitable emollient to soothe the skin and prevent or relieve dryness. Do, however, *avoid* the 'caine' products (e.g., the benzocaines). Although they may be cooling and lubricating, thus easing discomfort, they are common sensitizers, and could cause an allergic reaction.

See your doctor or dermatologist if vinegar, an emollient cream or the other simple measures just described fail to soothe the burn.

Severe sunburn

It's easier and more effective to prevent severe inflammation than to treat an already established reaction to a serious burn. If you're suffering from the results of overexposure to sunlamps or sunlight, *see a doctor immediately*. He or she may prescribe a short course of systemic corticosteroids, which may reduce a potentially severe burn.

The topical care of severe sunburn is usually to apply almost continuous cool compresses to the affected parts. Topical steroids may also be necessary, as well as pain-relieving medication (analgesics). Care may also sometimes be necessary to avoid pressure on the burned areas from bed linens, and careful observation is needed to detect any signs of bacterial infection.

Smoking and your skin

Tobacco is one of the two main culprits responsible for promoting wrinkling of skin (sun is the other). Smokers often develop well-defined wrinkles at the outer corners of their eyes ('crow's feet'). The skin on the back of their hands and neck tends to take on a cobblestone appearance and their complexion is inclined to be sallow.

Regular nicotine intake through smoking diminishes the skin's ability to heal itself. It has been clinically observed that among face-lift patients, heavy smokers were twelve times as liable to experience skin healing problems soon after surgery as non-smokers. To minimize risks, many plastic surgeons now advise their clients to stop smoking for several weeks before and after surgery.

Smoking destroys vitamin C and the B-complex vitamins, and also reduces vital oxygen supplies to the tissues. It contributes to premature ageing of the skin, manifested in such tell-tale signs as discoloration and wrinkling.

Studies done in the 1920s showed that the oxygen deprivation caused by smoking contributed to an acceleration of this ageing process.

Smoking a pack or more of cigarettes a day, over a long period of time, is especially injurious to the skin. It constricts, or tightens, the blood vessels that transport oxygen and other essential nutrients to the skin's cells. The skin then becomes prematurely wrinkled.

Oxygen, according to Paavo Airola, is the basic, most important nutrient of all living cells. The carbon monoxide from inhaled smoke (yours and someone else's) replaces the health- and life-giving oxygen in the blood-stream and tissues, and the results show.

Some years ago, a year-long study was made of visible damage from smoking. The results were striking: smokers between 40 and 50 years of age were as prominently wrinkled as non-smokers who were 20 years older!

Soap and water

Skin care experts agree that the first line of defence against problems is cleanliness. They suggest a regular bath or shower, without overuse of soap. They caution against the indiscriminate use of hot water and remind us that, even in winter, skin can dry out due to the cold and to forced-air heating in buildings.

According to one specialist in aesthetic medicine, soaps can contribute to skin dryness by emulsifying and removing the skin's natural oils. It takes the oil glands about six hours to restore the skin's normal acid mantle balance after a thorough cleansing with soap.

As already mentioned in Chapter 1, there are permanent resident flora on the skin. Far from being harmful, they may actually inhibit the growth of more virulent organisms, thus serving a natural protective function. In addition, a thin, liquid, lipid film, which provides even better protection, normally covers the skin. Unnecessary use of soap and water deprives skin of these two forms of protection.

Having said this, I feel I should tell you about the opinions of some dermatologists on this controversial subject of soap versus cleansing cream and lotions. Kenneth A. Arndt, M.D., Professor of Dermatology at Harvard Medical School, USA, has remarked that soap is not inherently harmful, and that some cleansing creams may in fact induce acneiform lesions (skin eruptions resembling acne). He recommends using a 'mild' soap or detergent bar, and keeping the number of washings per day to one or two — three at most — to minimize the drying effects of overwashing. To those persons who are obliged to wash their hands frequently (doctors and nurses, for example), Dr Arndt suggests using as little soap as possible and applying an emollient or a lubricant after washing.

Dr Zizmor has observed that researchers have tested 'everything from yogurt to sea mud' and have found nothing like good old soap and water to cut through oil and grime on acne-prone skin. Another expert's view is that while mild soaps and water can do the trick, as you age and your skin dries, you should probably switch to a cleansing lotion.

Cosmetologists tend to advocate the use of cleansers with a pH close to that of normal skin at its surface (6.8). They contend that soap, which is alkaline, removes this natural skin protection, leaving it susceptible to bacteria, dust and other pollutants, which can cause problems. One skin care authority recommends the use of naturally formulated cleansers or soaps with a pH of 5.5 to 7, to minimize skin irritation while promoting clean skin that looks and feels smooth. Another advises rinsing the face with cold water in the morning, and using a milk cleanser at night to free the skin of the day's accumulated pollutants and cosmetics.

Buying soaps

Always read the ingredient listing on packages of soap you plan to buy. Resorcinol is irritating to black skin. As a guideline, when purchasing soaps for acne-prone skin, 6 per cent of a surfactant ingredient (which strips the skin of oil and causes a mild peeling that unclogs pores) means that the soap is strong; 10 per cent means that it is *very strong*.

Clear and amber-coloured soaps are not, according to Dr Zizmor, better than opaque soaps. The reason why a soap is clear is that the manufacturer did not add the 'opacifier' that makes the product opaque. Dr Zizmor adds that clear versus opaque is simply a matter of aesthetics. Concerning pH balanced soaps, Dr Zizmor has this to say: Although an alkaline soap does reduce the skin's acidity, the protective 'acid mantle' will automatically restore itself in about forty-five minutes. Furthermore, while a pH balanced soap may be acidic in the bar or bottle, its pH changes the moment it is combined with water. Water has its own pH, and this varies from place to place.

If you wish to help nature restore the skin's pH balance after a soap and water wash, you can splash on a slightly acidic substance, such as apple cider vinegar or a mixture of lemon juice and water. Some dermatologists think it's a good idea to switch brands of soap occasionally. Always using the same soap can lessen its effectiveness and increase the chance of your developing an allergy to it.

Final notes on washing

Any skin cleansing routine should include washing the face twice daily, and also epiabrasion or exfoliation (described later in this chapter). Since each of us is a unique individual, however, it may be necessary to experiment to see what we find the most comfortable and effective. In addition, it is worth remembering that no routine will bring desired results unless it is carried out faithfully.

Oily (greasy) skin

Oily skin results from overactive oil glands. Oiliness varies with environmental conditions and with one's state of mind.

To determine if you have oily skin, rub a finger across your face, making sure that you're not sweating. If your skin feels slick, you probably have oily skin. If your skin feels constantly oily; if it feels oily less than one hour after having been washed or if it is noticeably shiny, it's likely to be very oily. You might also try this test: in the morning, blot your face with a paper tissue. If oil appears on the tissue, you have oily skin. If you have oily skin, it usually shows signs of oiliness half an hour or so after you awake in the morning.

As mentioned above, oily skin is caused by overactive sebaceous glands. This type of skin is more liable to eruptions than drier skin. If you have oily skin, however, you may have an advantage: as you grow older, you will most likely develop fewer wrinkles and look younger for a longer time than individuals with drier skin.

Caring for oily skin

There are several non-prescription products available to help care for oily skin, and you may need to experiment with a few before sticking with one that agrees with you, and which you enjoy using.

Here's a good basic daily routine for your skin type:

(1) Cleanse your skin with warm (*not* hot or cold) water and a good medicated soap. The purpose of washing with a specially formulated soap is not only to degrease and cleanse the skin, but also to promote a clearing up of any eruptions present.
(2) Lather and *gently* massage the soap into the skin, *except* the areas under the eyes. (If you have worn eye makeup, remove it with a special eye makeup remover before you wash your face.)
(3) Rinse the skin with warm water (hot water can break fragile capillaries in delicate skin; warm water is a better grease cutter than cold). Don't worry about leaving pores open).

When oil has accumulated on the skin between morning and evening and it's not possible to wash, here's what you can do.

Carry a travel-size container of astringent and some cotton wool puffs. Moisten a cotton puff with astringent and wipe away the oil. Towelettes premoistened with astringent are also available. If you don't wish to disturb your makeup, blot any surplus oil with linen tissues.

Blackheads (*open comedones*)

Blackheads appear when discoloured, dried sebum and dead cells plug the skin's excretory ducts. The dark colour at the top of blackheads is *not* dirt, and blackheads are *not* a result of being unclean. The dark colour is due to normal skin pigment (melanin).

Because blackheads extend 2 to 3 millimetres (⅛ inch) below the skin surface, washing alone won't get rid of them. It is *not* recommended to squeeze out blackheads, since this is painful and does not eliminate them (they re-form in a month or so). It is better to make *careful* use of a comedo extractor instead. This is a small metal tool used to push matter out of a pimple or pore. It is available at some chemists. However, it takes training and dexterity to use a comedo extractor without scarring the skin or causing infection, so before you use this instrument disinfect the affected areas with an astringent or rubbing alcohol. Better still, if the extraction of blackheads is done by a doctor, he or she will extract the plugs with a *sterilized* comedo extractor.

Caution

Please refrain from squeezing in the so-called 'Triangle of Death' area (extending from between the eyes to the corners of the mouth). The skin in this area covers a sinus cavity located beneath the brain. Veins in this triangle drain into this cavity. Should a serious infection develop, the results could prove fatal.

Epidermabrasion

Epidermabrasion, or 'epiabrasion' for short, is a procedure to remove the day's build-up of dead skin cells by gently 'sanding', or abrading, the skin surface. Simply washing with soap and water will not accomplish this, because dead cells are sticky and cling to the skin.

Any effective washing routine should include some form of epidermabrasion once a day. An acne face scrub is one way to epiabrade. If your skin is sensitive, however, epiabrade with soap and a soft-bristled complexion brush or other aid specially designed for this purpose.

Exfoliation

Exfoliation is, literally, scaling off dead tissue. Dead skin cells are chemically removed. Products formulated for this purpose are usually liquids, and are called by various names, such as 'clarifying', 'pore refining' or 'exfoliating' lotions. Their active ingredients are usually alcohol and salicylic acid, which is a peeling agent. These lotions are intended for use after a soap and water cleansing.

Other exfoliating agents include sea salt, yellow cornmeal and white sugar. Add a teaspoon of water to a small amount of any one of these ingredients, gradually increasing the moisture content until you obtain the consistency you desire. *Gently* massage your face and throat with the mixture, using your fingertips. Finish the procedure with a thorough *warm* water rinse.

Exfoliating lotions dissolve soap residue and that sticky, clogging layer of dead cells that make the complexion look dull.

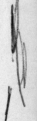

Exfoliation is one of the simplest methods of eliminating tiny wrinkles. Particularly likely to respond are the tiny wrinkles around the mouth and eyes. The rubbing action should be done perpendicular to the direction of the wrinkle. You might like to use a gently abrasive sponge and a cosmetic exfoliating agent. Remember to keep your touch very light.

Facials

A facial, sometimes called a 'professional cleansing' can prove very useful for blemished skin. However, you need to shop around for an establishment that will give you your money's worth. Properly carried out, a facial can be very relaxing.

Note. Don't use this method is you have acne.

An at-home facial

You can do your own facial at home by observing the following steps:

(1) *Washing.* Wash your face and pat it dry. *Do not* apply a skin toner, astringent or moisturizer.

(2) *Steaming.* Steaming softens the skin and oil plugs, so that these can be removed without difficulty. Steam the face as follows:

— Boil some water. Pour the boiling water into a large bowl. Add herbs, such as 'Swiss Kriss', which is a laxative tea containing over a dozen detoxifying herbs. It is available at some chemists and health food stores. It is also available in tablet form. (Two tablespoons of herbs or one tablet will suffice.) Alternatively, you may immerse a few chamomile tea bags in the bowl of water.

— Place the bowl of water on a heat-proof surface. Sit so you can conveniently lean over the bowl without being burned. Drape a towel over your head to make an improvised 'steam tent'. Steam your face for 5 to 8 minutes, or as long as the steam lasts.

(3) Deep pore cleansing. The next step of the facial is deep pore cleansing, or exfoliation (see the previous section). Another exfoliant (exfoliating agent) you can make, *before you steam your face*, is a mixture of one teaspoon each of crushed oats, cornmeal, plain yogurt and honey. Gently massage your face and neck for 1 minute with this mixture (or another exfoliant of your choice). Use slow, circular motions, emphasizing the upward strokes. Finish the procedure with a *warm* water rinse. pat the skin dry with a soft, absorbent towel.

(4) *Applying a mask.* Next comes application of a facial mask. This is a thick mixture that is spread on the face and allowed to dry. While drying, it draws remaining impurities from the pores and tightens them. When it is removed, it takes with it impurities and dead cells.

The mask is usually left on for 10 to 20 minutes before it is removed. This period is an excellent time to lie on a Slant Board and relax (see Chapter 6).

Chemists and health food stores carry a variety of facial masks, but you can make some at home:

— Whip two egg whites to form stiff peaks. Add the juice of half a lemon and gently mix the ingredients together.

Spread the mask on your face and leave it on for 20 minutes. Rinse it off with tepid water.

— Mix about ⅓ cup of almond meal with enough witch hazel to make a paste. Apply the mask to your face, particularly to areas with blackheads. Leave the paste on for 20 minutes (or until it begins to crack). Rinse it off with tepid water.

Notes on facial ingredients:

— Almond meal is slightly abrasive.

— Egg white is drying.

— Fuller's earth (a dry clay, available in health food stores) has natural 'drawing out' abilities.

— Honey is moisturizing.

— Oatmeal is soothing.

— Tannic acid (found in regular tea) is soothing.

(5) *Completing the facial.* To complete your facial, apply a skin toner, an eye oil and a moisturizer. It is a good idea to keep the skin free of makeup for at least 2 hours following a facial.

Most of us live in polluted environments. Periodic deeper-than-usual cleansings can remove pollutants, grease and grime and prevent their build-up. A properly executed facial can give the skin a fresh start and help it look and feel wonderful.

Dry skin

If your skin is dry or tends to be dry, you need to moisturize it regularly with a suitable lotion or cream. Your selection of moisturizer is important. An effective skin care product for this purpose should contain such nutrients as vitamins A and E, UVA and UVB filters for protection from sun, and EFAs, which play a vital role in the lipid (fat) structure of the epidermis. EFAs help to maintain the skin's moisture balance, thus preventing undue water loss across this protective barrier with which nature has furnished us.

With an intelligent choice of moisturizer and with faithful use, drying of the skin, which leads to loss of elasticity and consequent premature ageing, can be kept to a minimum.

Remember to apply your dry skin lotion or cream within 3 minutes of bathing or showering (or washing the face and hands) to take advantage of the water trapped by the skin. Of the two or three daily applications of skin cream or lotion you need, the one immediately after the shower or bath is the most important for capturing and holding moisture and reducing or discouraging cracking and chapping. You might also try applying a bath oil directly to the skin, rather than using it in the bathtub where it becomes too dilute for effectiveness.

According to one professor of dermatology, the use of bath oils and/or special 'superfatted' soaps to counteract dryness often provides the user with a false sense of security. It may encourage excessive cleansing, with consequent aggravation of the dry skin.

Persons with with a dry skin problem would also be wise to keep the temperature in their home somewhat on the cool side and use soft, non-irritating bed clothing, keeping these to a minimum.

Itching (pruritus)

Itching is a symptom of irritation of the nerve endings that transmit pain stimuli. Severe itching may be an early sign of diabetes or cancer, or a liver or thyroid disorder. Other factors exciting or contributing to itching include drug reactions, stress, pregnancy, or menopause.

In attempting to treat itching, the offending agent must be identified and dealt with. If you suspect that a medication you're taking may be generating the itch, *check with your doctor* to see if you can stop using it.

Good hygiene is important, but if your skin tends to be dry, avoid frequent cleansing with soap and water. Take short, warm showers instead of prolonged hot baths. Also, stay away from perfumed soaps. Perfume is one of the most common allergy-causing substances. Often it serves no practical purpose, and it does add considerably to the cost of the product.

My family tends to be sensitive to highly perfumed products. I once used a lotion — one of the *Efamolia* range of skin care products — to massage my older son's neck and shoulders to help ease a tension headache. I waited for him to comment on the smell. I was pleasantly surprised when he voiced no objection. This lotion, in fact, contains ingredients I have suggested earlier in this chapter as desirable for fabulous skin. The EPO in the product has such a delicate fragrance that even the most sensitive nostrils would not be offended.

If you have itching skin, be careful as well of using deodorant soaps (see section on sun and skin). Soaking in water to which a packet of colloidal oatmeal has been added is often an effective anti-itch treatment. Colloidal oatmeal bars (a soap alternative) are also very soothing, and my young sons find them pleasant and effective.

Do avoid sudden water temperature changes if you have an itching problem. Dry yourself ever so gently with a soft, non-irritating towel and put on soft, loose-fitting garments.

If your itching persists, do *consult your doctor.*

Sometimes, a soothing lotion such as calamine, is useful to bring temporary relief. Do, however, steer clear of creams, lotions or sprays that contain local anaesthetics. They can further irritate the skin and worsen the itching.

Here, finally, is information of some specific types of itching, or *pruritus*, which will be indicated by the letter 'p'.

p. ani	Itching around the anus. It may be due to haemorrhoids (piles) or to contact with soaps and detergents that remain in inadequately laundered underclothing.
p. essential	Itching without a noticeable skin lesion (diseased part of body).
p. hiemalis (winter itch)	Itching that occurs in cold weather. It is aggravated by cooling of the skin.
p. symptomatic	Itching that is a symptom of some other disorder.
p. vulvae	Severe itching of the external female genitals. It is often an early sign of diabetes; it can also indicate vaginitis (inflammation of the vagina).

For information on rashes, please see Chapter 5.

Sex and the skin

Although some skin specialists scoff at the notion that sexual activity is wonderful for the skin, others are not as sceptical. One believer has remarked that sex, having the potential of a marvellous tension reliever, actually makes skin glow.

As sexual excitement intensifies, the heart pumps blood faster and breathing accelerates. Consequently, a richer supply of blood reaches all the body's billions of cells, thus providing health-giving oxygen and other nutrients. At the same time, with each exhalation, waste products are effectively eliminated through the lungs. That is why, at the peak of sexual activity, a blush-like colour often appears on the skin of the face, neck and chest. That is why, too, some individuals' complexions take on such a radiance when they're enjoying an exciting, satisfying sexual relationship.

The endocrine glands, which regulate so many of the body's vital functions, are also beneficially stimulated during sex. Through them, skin, hair and nails (and other structures as well) receive wonderful benefits.

Skin. Blood vessels of the skin relax and allow more blood and heat to reach the surface. This results in an improved supply of nutrients and, even though you can't see it, more oil and moisture to the pores. There is also better moisture retention to discourage drying out of the skin, leaving it soft, silky and sensuous to touch.

Hair. Especially if you're lying flat (without a pillow) during sex, the scalp and hair receive a better supply of nutrient-rich blood. This helps to strengthen the hair 'roots', prevents abnormal hair fall and gives protection against brittleness and split ends. Hair thrives and looks fuller and more lustrous.

Nails. Because of a general improvement in the blood circulation during sexual activity, nails tend to grow faster, become smoother, stronger and shinier, and are less prone to break and split.

Eyes. During orgasm, the tiny muscles around the eyes are exercised in a very natural way, and this counteracts the tendency to upper and lower eyelid droop and to puffy skin around the eyes.

Jaws. During orgasm, the muscles around the jaws are exercised,

with a consequent improvement in muscle tone. This helps
prevent a double chin and furrows at the corners of the mouth.
Neck. As sexual excitement peaks, the muscles at the front of the
neck receive a therapeutic stretch (provided your head is not on
a pillow). This promotes firmness and smoothness of the throat.

Oleda Baker and Bill Gale (see Bibliography) have offered helpful
hints to discourage inhibition of the beauty orgasm. Here are
some of them:
— Keep your bedroom environment relaxing and inviting.
— Wear attractive, freshly laundered clothing at bed-time.
— Avoid monotony. Be flexible with regard to time, place and
technique.
— Show warmth and affection not only during sexual intimacy,
but at others times as well.

Skin in pregnancy

Most of the changes to the skin (as well as to the hair and nails)
that occur in pregnancy are due to altered hormonal levels. The
thought is comforting though, that with adequate nutrition, rest
and exercise, these features should return to normal a few months
after baby is born.

Freckles and birthmarks tend to darken in pregnancy. Some
women also develop *melasma gravidarum* (discoloration of skin in
pregancy), or a 'mask of pregnancy' — this is a patchy pigmentation that may appear on the forehead, cheeks and elsewhere,
and often includes darkening of the skin on the upper lip. If you
develop melasma, you should avoid the sun, since it darkens this
'mask'. You should also regularly use a sunscreen with an SPF of
15 (see the section on sunscreens earlier in this chapter).

Do not bleach any increased skin pigmentation. If you do, you
risk sensitization from certain ingredients in the bleaching agents.
Most women who develop melasma can expect it to disappear a
few weeks after the baby's birth. Any increase in facial or body
hair, caused by altered levels of hormones in pregnancy, will also
usually vanish.

There is a tendency to itchiness during pregnancy. This can

usually be relieved by using colloidal oatmeal in the bath water and a moisturizing skin lotion afterwards.

Scars formed at this time are apt to be darker than usual and more noticeable. This isn't because pregnant women scar more easily, but because of an increase in the level of a hormone that intensifies pigmentation. Pregnant women should therefore be especially careful when shaving. They should also refrain from picking at pimples (everyone should).

In pregnancy, the eccrine glands produce more sweat than usual, while the apocrine glands secrete less. An increased production of oil, which causes some women's complexions to glow, and which produces pimples in others, also accounts for little bumps that sometimes appear in the dark pigmented area surrounding the nipples (areolae).

Striae, which are purple or red stretch marks, appear on the breasts and abdomen of about 80 per cent of pregnant women. These are more likely the result of increased hormonal levels than actual stretching of the skin. Although doctors usually suggest that women cream or oil their body so as to control these marks, it has not been proven whether this is effective or not. The striae do eventually fade in the months following delivery. An oil or cream may be used, however, to relieve itching. It should be massaged into the skin very gently.

Blood circulatory changes may cause spider veins to appear on the face, neck and chest. These usually disappear shortly after delivery.

Finally, be wary of vitamin preparations specially formulated for pregnant women. If you have been prescribed one that contains iodine, discuss it with your doctor. This mineral can trigger an outbreak of acne.

Women who keep themselves in tip-top condition before and during pregnancy tend to recover more fully and quickly from childbirth than those who have not adequately cared for themselves. If you wish more in-depth information on looking and feeling good all over, and on keeping healthy during pregnancy and afterwards, please read the updated edition of my book *Easy Pregnancy with Yoga* (Thorsons, 1991).

Time of Month

When a girl begins to menstruate, her periods may be irregular and her oil glands may produce much more oil than her skin needs. Even when menstrual periods are established, oiliness and blemishes can occur in response to hormonal imbalances during 'that time of month'.

In most women who suffer from premenstrual syndrome (PMS), skin disorders are not an uncommon problem. There is an increased tendency to acne during the premenstrual week, and there may also be unexplained bruising. In addition, allergies — which are thought to be associated with PMS — may be more noticeable. Probably the worst effect of these signs and symptoms is the lowering of a woman's morale. These blemishes and other undesirable conditions usually clear up, however, once the period has started.

The advice usually given for dealing with teenage acne is also applicable to premenstrual skin disorders. It includes using a mildly medicated soap and avoiding fatty foods such as potato chips and other deep-fried foods. It's a good idea, too, to take extra care of the skin a few days before you expect its condition to worsen: adhere to a wholesome diet, drink extra water or mineral water and exercise regularly, preferably out of doors. To camouflage particularly noticeable spots, you may wish to use a 'masking' cream, which should be washed off at night. After drying the skin, you can then apply antiseptic ointment, using a light touch.

Some wonderful results have been obtained from the use of evening primrose oil (see Chapter 4) in combination with zinc. If acne or other skin eruptions persist, however, do *see a doctor*.

Generally, women who are conscientious about maintaining a high standard of health tend to encounter fewer menstrual and premenstrual problems than women who don't. I have gone into various aspects of self-care, including diet, exercise and stress management in my book entitled *Pain-Free Periods* (Thorsons, 1986).

Dry brushing

Dry brushing is a health-promoting technique for helping to remove dead cells from the skin surface and for improving the blood supply and nourishment to the skin. It is done with a special brush or mitt, made of natural hemp fibre, which is available at health food stores.

Dry brushing is usually done in the morning before showering. Start with the right foot, then proceed to the abdomen, brushing with a circular motion from the lower right to the lower left side and round again. Follow with the right and then the left hand and arm; afterwards do the chest, making a figure-eight around the breasts.

Taking the brush's straps, brush the bottom next, using a back-and-forth motion, then moving upward to the waistline. Finish with the upper back, until it feels pleasantly warm.

Ten steps to healthier skin

Here's a sort of checklist I've devised to help you attain and maintain the best possible skin conditions. It's especially useful for very busy persons with demanding schedules.

Make a copy of it and place it where you can refer to it regularly. It will alert you to areas of skin care you may have been neglecting, so that you may rectify these to keep your skin looking fabulous. If you want to review each step in detail, refer to the chapter number given in brackets.

1. *Diet*. Regularly eat wholesome food (3). Drink plenty of water to prevent dehydration.
2. *Elimination*. Regular elimination of waste products from the body is vital to skin health (7).
3. *Exercise*. Regular outdoor and indoor exercise is important (7).
4. *Stress management*. Daily relaxation and adequate sleep are two invaluable components of any stress management programme (6).
5. *Reduce smoking and alcohol and caffeine intake* (3,9).
6. *Hygiene*:
   — Gentle cleansing with a mild soap or with a non-alkaline soap alternative.

— Brisk towelling with a soft, absorbent towel, to help dispose of dead surface cells and stimulate cell renewal. Use firm light strokes on the face and be especially gentle on the areas around the eyes; or simply blot surplus moisture with your towel.

— Consider the occasional use of a natural face pack. Lie on a Slant Board while the pack does it work (6).

7. *Protection*:

— Effective protection from the sun (9).

— Regular use of moisturizers with protective ingredients to provide an invisible barrier against the potentially harmful effects of environmental irritants.

8. *Repair.* Regular use of wisely selected skin care products with natural ingredients to help repair damaged cells and to restore the skin's integrity.

9. *Nourishment.* Regular use of intelligently selected skin care products with natural ingredients such as EPO (evening primrose oil) and vitamins A and E. These are external complements to the nutrients obtained internally through a wholesome diet, and together represent total skin care needs (5, 9).

10. Thirty Days To Stronger Nails

In 1979, a 55-year-old woman with a six-month history of dry, gritty eyes and brittle nails which tended to split when manicured, was treated with a product rich in essential fatty acids (EFAs). Her eye condition gradually improved and, after one month, she reported that her nails had become normal.

In the same year, an older woman with an eight-month history of dry, gritty eyes, and a six-month history of nails that split and broke, was similarly treated. Within a month her eyes improved and shortly thereafter her nails became normal.

In 1980, a 53-year-old woman who had a longstanding problem with tear secretion was treated with the same product as the other two women just mentioned. In only one month her eyes improved, as did her nails, which had been brittle and splitting for half a year.

Medical doctors and skin specialists advise people with nail problems such as these to avoid frequent wetting and drying of the hands, and recommend the application of emollient creams to soothe and soften them. This type of treatment is not always practicable, however. Nurses, for example, are required to wash their hands frequently while on the job, often with anti-bacterial agents which are, in the long term unkind to the hands and fingernails. Moreover, local application of creams and ointments does not always bring expected results.

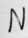

The three women mentioned were treated systemically with *Efamol* evening primrose oil, that is, they took it internally, in the form of capsules. This therapy, bringing the wonderful results it did in just thirty days, is more than a little persuasive that a nutritional approach to the problem of brittle and splitting nails may be of substantial and lasting value. It clearly suggests that these disorders may be, at least in part, due to an underlying EFA (essential fatty acid) deficiency. It also indicates that supplementation with a clinically well-tested brand of evening primrose oil could set right the probable deficiency.

As I was writing the script for this book, a stubborn fingernail problem I had had for over a year apparently began to resolve itself. I had brought home from a visit to London two jars of moisturizing cream and a bottle of lotion — a range of skin care products that had just come on the market. The products contain natural ingredients, including *Efamol* evening primrose oil (EPO). Diligently every morning and evening I used my hands to apply the creams or lotion to various parts of my body and to massage them in. Afterwards, I also massaged my hands with the lotion. In only one month, the middle fingernail of my right hand — the problem nail — had knit together again. It had split and would not mend despite various topical and systemic treatments.

Was it mere coincidence, I asked myself, that these products had succeeded, where others had failed, because of their EPO content?

A primrose by any other name
Not all oils extracted from the seeds of all evening primrose plants are alike. In fact, only the products that have been subjected to rigorous testing and stringent quality control are worthy of ingestion or application to your skin. The crucial ingredient in EPO is gamma-linolenic acid, or GLA. It must be present in sufficient quality to be effective. If it isn't, then you're wasting your money.

The reasons why a particular brand of EPO may seem 'expensive' compared with other brands are basically because of the high cost of clinical trials and research, as well as high quality control to which it is subjected. The trials in which a product is involved are very costly to conduct. They have to be financed by the product itself, and this is precisely why most firms marketing evening primrose oil do not carry out such trials.

Getting to the root

If you look back at Chapter 1, you will be reminded that the deeper skin layers house important structures, which include nerve endings, blood vessels and fat and connective tissue elements. You will recall, too, that it is by way of the blood-stream that all the body's cells receive nutrients that keep them healthy.

Fingernails and toenails are very similar to human hair. Both structures begin deep inside the skin; both rely on body processes such as the circulation of blood for nourishment, growth and health. In fact, the chemical components of the nails are similar to those of the hair.

When a reliable source of EFAs is taken into the body, it reaches the tissues deficient in them, provided there is nothing to block its pathway. Evening primrose oil, as a practical and superb source of GLA, is not subject to the many potential blockages to which some other EFA sources are exposed. It's therefore a smooth passage from GLA to PGE1.

Gelatin for nails

It's a fallacy that gelatin strengthens and helps repair nails. Yet many people, professionals included, cling to this myth. It is true that fingernails are made of protein. But gelatin lacks so many essential protein building-blocks (amino acids) that it actually inhibits healing. Moreover, it supplies such an excess of glycine (the simplest of amino acids) that it can be toxic when added to an otherwise adequate diet.

There is absolutely no sound scientific evidence to support claims that gelatin (or calcium for that matter) can help produce healthy nails. Adequate nutrition is what's best for the formation of any body tissue, nails included. Team that up with proper local nail care and you have the best possible chance for healthy, attractive nails.

Local nail care

Proper nail care is a many-faceted affair, involving not only a systemic, or 'whole body' approach, but also a topical, or local one. In the former, we look after the nails from inside the body for, like other tissues, nails rely on good nutrition for good health and this starts from within. In the latter aspect of care, we focus attention on the nails from the outside.

Here is a basic, no-nonsense specimen guide for the care of the nails. It takes only minutes and is therefore practical for today's busy person with little time for complex nail care rituals.

Manicure

The best time for a manicure is after a bath or shower. If this isn't convenient, wash your hands well prior to your nail care routine.

1. Clean under the nails, gently, so as not to break the skin where it's attached to the nails. It's easy for yeasts and bacteria ('germs') to enter tissues through skin breaks. Infection may then result, or the nail plate may separate from the underlying skin. For this purpose, it's best to use a soft nail brush or an orangewood stick to coax away dirt adhering stubbornly to the nails.

2. Lovingly dry and buff each nail with a soft towel, paying special attention to the nail groove where the nail meets the skin of the finger. If you allow, say, three seconds per nail, this takes only half a minute.

An alternative way of buffing the nails is to use a good quality chamois buffer, buffing the nails gently in one direction only. Try to do this once a week, or at least once a month, as nail buffing promotes blood circulation to the fingers and imparts a healthy lustre to the nails.

3. Remove nail polish carefully with a mild nail polish remover. Rinse the hands and dry them well. If your nails are very weak, file them first (see step 4) before removing polish, to minimize the chances of damaging them.

4. Trim the fingernails if necessary. Most manicurists suggest nail clippers, rather than scissors which can crack or split the nails. Next, smooth the nails with an emery board, *filing in one direction only*. Interestingly, some manicurists consider even emery boards too abrasive, and encourage the use of a 'diamond dust' file instead.

5. Apply polish if you so desire, and let it dry thoroughly. Beauty

experts suggest that you stick to more subdued, neutral colours if you keep your nails short, leaving brighter colours to individuals with long nails.

Authorities recommend the use of nail enamel, especially in winter, as it helps seal in moisture and protect nails from dry environments. They also advocate shorter nails at this time of year to discourage breaking.

6. Generously cream your fingers, hands, wrists, elbows and forearms with a good quality, non-greasy lotion. I suggest a brand containing natural ingredients such as evening primrose oil and vitamins A and E, as well as an effective sunscreen.

Hand and fingertips
Your hands are constantly on display and can enhance or mar the impression you make on others.

— Develop the habit of wearing cotton-lined rubber gloves when washing dishes or clothes or doing household chores. Use gardening gloves for outdoor jobs. Alkali soaps and detergents disrupt the natural acid mantle on the skin's surface. This 'mantle' helps ward off bacterial infection, and its removal sets the scene for 'dishpan' hands and skin rashes.

— Generously apply hand cream to hands and fingernails after every wash or soaking in water.

— Train yourself to use the 'pads' of your fingers rather than your fingertips or fingernails when using the telephone dial, typing, untying packages, etc.

— Resist the urge to tap impatiently with your fingertips when you feel under stress. Try to find something more constructive for your hands to do, or practise slow, deep rhythmic breathing instead. Also curb the tendency to bite or pick at nails, or flick one against another. These are bad habits which promote nail damage.

— Practise *The Flower* exercise (see Chapter 7).

— Generously apply your favourite skin cream or lotion to your hands, slip on a pair of cotton gloves and relax on a Slant Board (see Chapter 6) for 20 minutes at least once a week (twice a week is better).

— Your real nails, however inadequate they may seem to you, are probably better than artificial nails. Frequent use of false nails will cause waterlogging of the real ones, weaken them and cause them to deteriorate. Even short nails can look very attractive if properly manicured.

— Since the cuticle lies so near the nail matrix (the nail's 'manufacturing plant'), any but the gentlest of cuticle care can injure this delicate and important structure, perhaps permanently. So, *treat your cuticle very gently indeed. Don't cut it. Don't* push any instrument under it. *Do* keep it well moisturized to prevent it from cracking. Health food stores sell specially formulated creams to nourish and strengthen cuticles. Many contain a variety of essential nutrients, including the mineral silica, which is essential for strong nails.

— Wear lined gloves outdoors. Leather tends to absorb essential oils from the skin.

Nail wrapping

Naturally, it's best to encourage the growth and maintenance of strong, problem-free nails through healthful living. There are times, though, when time is of the essence, and you may have to resort to a temporary expedient. Nail wrapping may then be something worth looking into.

Nail wrapping is a procedure some manicurists suggest for reinforcing weak nails that tend to split, break or tear. There are basically two types of wraps: liquid and solid. The former are essentially nail polishes containing nylon fibres. You can apply them first in one direction then in the other for extra strength. If you can't manage to have a solid wrap, then liquid nail wraps are better than nothing.

Solid wraps offer more protection than their liquid counterparts. They come in nail-wrap kits, which are available at some chemists, and they usually contain pre-cut wraps (silk or other material), quick-bonding nail glue, a buffer and instructions for wrapping.

How to wrap a nail

(1) Smooth the unpolished nail with the buffer.

(2) Apply the nail glue to cover the damaged part of the nail and surrounding area. Use the glue sparingly, and follow the instructions for its use very carefully. Avoid the skin and cuticles.

(3) Before this fast-drying glue sets, apply a piece of wrap to the tip of the nail, allowing the material to extend over the free edge. Adjust placement of the wrap, if necessary, using an orangewood stick. Hold the wrap securely in place to prevent it from slipping.

(4) Apply another coat of nail glue over the wrap, for added reinforcement, ensuring that it has been completely saturated.

(5) Let the glue dry completely.

(6) Trim and/or file surplus wrapping material from the free edge of the nail.

(7) Buff the dried surface of the wrap until it is flush with the nail and no line of demarcation is visible. The entire surface should feel smooth.

(8) You may again apply nail glue and allow it to dry.

(9) Buff the dried surface until it is flush with the natural nail.

(10) Apply nail polish, as you would in a regular manicure: a base coat, nail colour and a top coat are suggested to complete the nail wrapping. Let each coat dry thoroughly before applying the next.

Removing polish from a wrapped nail

— Use a non-acetone remover; it won't loosen the nail wrap.

Whenever you change nail polish, first check carefully to make sure that the wrap is still intact, especially at the corners of the nail. If you find loose areas, apply nail glue under and over these, let the glue dry thoroughly, buff, and then apply polish.

Taking off the wrap

A nail wrap should last until the nail has grown out. Should you decide to take the wrap off, however, first remove the polish from the nail, then buff the wrap with a nail buffer until you reach the natural nail. Alternatively, you can use a solvent manufactured for this purpose. This tends to dry the nail, though.

In either case, soak the nail in olive oil after removing the wrap, so as to help restore its suppleness. If the nails seems soft or weak, you can apply one coat of liquid fibre wrap horizontally, allow it to dry for a minute or two, then apply a second coat vertically and allow that to dry. This gives reinforcement to the nail. After about five minutes, apply a base coat and nail polish.

It's not a bad idea to let a professional manicurist do your first nail wrap. Once you see the right way to do it, you can more confidently do it yourself at home.

Nail hardeners and false nails

Nail strengthening products are, as the name implies, formulated to do just that. Nail hardeners, used often, will harden nails — but with significant risk. There's a chance that they can cause *onycholysis*, a condition in which the nail plate separates from the nail bed. They may also discolour the nail plate or cause bleeding under it.

Artificial nails may prove a boon if you have an important function to attend at short notice. Be aware, however, that the adhesive used to apply them can occasionally cause sensitization reactions in some people.

Pedicure

1. Like the manicure, pedicure is best done after a soak in the bathtub or after a shower. Otherwise, immerse the feet in a basin of warm water for several minutes, cleanse them thoroughly as in the manicure just described, and dry them well with a soft towel paying particular attention to those areas where skin meets nail.
2. Remove nail polish. Rinse and dry the toes.
3. Cut the toenails *straight across*, keeping the nail edges level with the tips of the toes. The free nail edge should be at right angles to the lateral (side) edges. If the nails are highly convex, cutting away the sides actually encourages their penetration into the lateral grooves.
4. For a smooth finish, file them with an emery board so that no pointed edges remain.
5. Buff the nails and leave them unpolished; or apply polish and let it dry thoroughly.

6. Generously massage the feet with your favourite skin cream or lotion, paying special attention to the heels and balls of the feet, where skin tends to become hard and rough. Also treat the knees in the same way. Remember to use a skin care product rich in natural ingredients such as evening primrose oil and vitamins A and E.

Toe and foot notes

Although feet may be concealed a good deal of the time, they are usually on view in summer. Even when you aren't preparing to bare your feet to the public eye, however, pampering them is wonderfully restorative to the whole body.

— For a superb beauty treatment, apply a good quality skin cream or lotion to the feet, put on cotton socks and lie on a Slant Board for 20 minutes (see Chapter 6) at least once a week.

— Practise the *Legs Up* exercise (see Chapter 6) at the end of each day's work.

— Practise the *Dog Stretch* (described in Chapter 7) at least every other day.

— Wear proper fitting shoes with sensible heels. Be particularly prudent in your choice of footwear if you jog frequently or play one of the racquet games such as tennis. If your shoes are too short, your toenails will be subjected to trauma which can lead to separation of the nail from the bed, or to damage to the nail matrix itself.

— Walk barefoot on grass or a sandy beach whenever you can.

— Women, give *him* a pedicure as a special treat. Men, do the same for *her*. Oriental wisdom has it that the feet are the way to the heart!

GLOSSARY

Acid mantle	Refers to the acid state of normal skin, which helps protect it from penetration by harmful bacteria.
Adrenal glands	Two endocrine glands located on top of the kidneys.
Adrenalin (epinephrine)	A hormone secreted by the medullae (middle part) of the adrenal glands.
Aerobic	Living only in the presence of oxygen. Aerobic exercise is exercise during which the energy needed is supplied by the oxygen inhaled.
Aesthetician	Professionally licensed cosmetic skin specialist.
Allergen	Any substance that produces an allergy.
Allergy	Altered reaction of body tissues to an allergen.
Alopecia	Deficiency of hair. Baldness.
Alpha-linolenic acid	Same as linolenic acid.
Amino acid	The end-product of protein digestion. Protein building-block.
Anaemia	Deficiency in quantity or quality of red blood cells.
Anaesthetic	An agent causing insensibility

	to pain or touch.
Anagen	The growing stage of hair development.
Analgesic	A remedy that relieves pain.
Antagonist	Something that counteracts the action of something else.
Antibiotic	A substance that destroys or inhibits the growth of micro-organisms.
Antibody	Specific substance formed in the body, which counteracts the effects of bacterial poisons.
Antihistamine	A drug that counteracts the action of histamine.
Antioxidant	A substance that slows down the destructive effects of oxygen or other substances.
Antiscorbutic	An agent effective against scurvy, a vitamin C deficiency disease.
Apocrine glands	Sweat glands located only in hairy areas of the body, such as the groins and armpits.
Arachidonic acid	A polyunsaturated fatty acid.
Astringent	An agent that has a constricting or binding effect.
Atopy	A word used to describe a group of diseases of an allergic nature.
Atrophy	A wasting due to lack of nutrition. A diminution in the size of a cell, tissue, organ or part.
Bacteria (sing. bacterium)	A general name given to minute vegetable organisms which live on organic matter.
Bactericidal	Capable of killing bacteria, e.g.,

	disinfectants, great heat or sunlight.
Balm	A soothing or healing ointment.
Basal	Pertaining to the base of anything; of primary importance.
Bioflavonoids	A group of nutrients associated with vitamin C. Also called vitamin P.
Blackhead	Discoloured dried sebum plugging an excretory duct of the skin. Also known as an open comedo (plural, comedones). The black part is caused by melanin, *not* by dirt.
Capillary	Literally, 'hair-like'. Capillaries are minute vessels connecting an artery and a vein. They may also be found in the lymphatic system.
Carcinogenic	Cancer-producing.
Carcinoma	A malignant epithelial tumour. Cancer.
Carob flour	A fine, light-brown powder that looks like cocoa or chocolate. Made from the ground seed pods of a Mediterranean tree. Also called carob powder.
Carotene	A yellow pigment found in various plant and animal tissues. It is a precursor of vitamin A.
Catagen	Refers to the intermediate state of the hair growth cycle, between the anagen and telogen stages.
Catalyst	A substance that speeds up the rate of a chemical reaction without itself being permanently

altered in the reaction.

Co-factors
Agents that facilitate chemical reactions (e.g., enzymes, minerals and vitamins).

Collagen
A fibrous insoluble protein found in connective tissue, including skin. It represents about 30 per cent of the total body protein.

Comedo (pl., comedones)
See Blackhead.

Corium
See Dermis.

Cornified
Refers to the conversion of squamous (i.e., scaly) epithelial cells into hard material, e.g. hair.

Cutaneous
Pertaining to the skin.

Cuticle
The epidermis, or external layer of skin.

Cuticle of hair shaft
A single layer of clear cells which forms the outer layer of a hair.

Cuticle of the nail
The skin growing onto the nail from the nail folds.

Cyanosis
A bluish appearance, usually of the skin and mucous membranes.

Dehydration
Occurs when the body is deprived of water or when there is excessive fluid loss.

Delta-6-desaturase (D6D)
An enzyme vital for the conversion of linoleic acid to gamma-linolenic acid (GLA).

Dermatitis
Inflammation of the skin.

Dermatologist
A physician who specializes in diseases of the skin.

Dermis
The true skin, which lies under the epidermis. The corium.

Dihomogamma-linolenic acid (DGLA)	A fatty acid; found in human milk and some organ meats.
Distal	Situated away from the centre of the body or point of origin. Opposite of proximal.
Diuretic	An agent that increases the secretion of urine.
DNA (deoxy-ribonucleic acid)	The nucleic acid that transmits information from parent to offspring. The chemical basis of heredity. The carrier of genetic information for almost all organisms.
Eccrine glands	Glands that secrete sweat.
Ectoderm	The outer layer of cells in a developing embryo.
Eczema	An acute or chronic inflammatory condition of the skin, generally non-contagious.
Eczematous	Affected with, or resembling eczema.
EFAs	Essential fatty acids.
Elastin	A protein substance found in the dermis; gives skin elasticity.
Eleidin	A translucent compound, found in the stratum lucidum of the epidermis, from which keratin is formed.
Embryo	The young of any organism in an early stage of development; in humans, between second and eighth weeks inclusive.
Embryonic	Pertaining to an embryo.
Emollient	An agent that soothes and softens a part of the body when applied locally.

Endocrine gland	A gland whose secretion (hormone) flows directly into the blood-stream and is circulated to all parts of the body.
Enzyme	A complex protein that is capable of bringing about chemical changes in other substances without being changed itself.
Epidermis	The outer layer, or cuticle, of the skin.
Epithelial	Refers to the epithelium.
Epithelium	The layer of cells forming the epidermis.
EPO	Evening primrose oil.
Eruption	Literally, a breaking out, especially applied to the appearance of a skin lesion (local diseased part), such as a rash.
Erythema	Reddening of the skin.
Essential fatty acids (EFAs)	Fatty acids required by the body for vital functions which the body cannot make, and which must be supplied by food.
Exacerbate	To aggravate symptoms.
Excretory	Pertaining to the elimination of waste products from the body.
Exocrine glands	Glands whose secretion reaches an epithelial surface either directly or through a duct. Sebaceous glands are examples of exocrine glands.
Fatty acids	Major building-blocks of the fats in foods and human bodies; important energy sources.
Follicle (hair)	The sheath in which a hair grows.

Frontalis muscle (occipito frontalis)	A muscle covering the skull. It runs from above the eyebrows to the back of the head and controls the movements of the scalp and face.
Gamma-linolenic acid (GLA)	A substance made from linoleic acid by healthy cells. Also found in evening primrose oil and human milk.
Haemoglobin	The colouring matter of red blood cells.
Hangnail	Partly detached piece of skin at the root of a fingernail.
Histamine	A chemical substance produced when tissues are injured.
Hormone	A chemical substance generated in one organ and carried by the blood to another in which it excites activity. A secretion of endocrine (ductless) glands.
Humectant	A moistening agent.
Hyper-	A prefix meaning above, excessive, or beyond.
Hypertrophy	Excessive thickening of a part or organ through the increase of its own tissues.
Hypo-	A prefix indicating less than, below, or under.
Hypothalamus	Part of the brain recognized as being important in emotion.
Imbrications	Overlapping, as of tiles or fish scales.
Immune system	The body's natural defences against disease.

Integument	Literally, a covering. Usually refers to the skin.
Intravenous	Within or into a vein.
Jaundice	A yellow discoloration of the skin.
Keratin	An extremely tough protein substance in hair, skin and nails.
Laxative	A food or chemical substance which helps to loosen the bowels to counteract constipation.
Lesion	An infected patch, as in a skin disease.
Linolenic acid (LNA)	An essential fatty acid. It cannot be made by the body and must therefore be supplied by food.
Lipid	A word used to describe fats, oils and other fatty substances.
Lymph	The fluid from the blood which has passed through capillary walls to supply nutrients to tissue cells.
Lymphatic system	A system of vessels and glands involved in transporting lymph from the tissues to the bloodstream.
Malignant	A term applied to any disease of a virulent and fatal nature.
Matrix	The basic substance from which something is made.
Melanin	The pigment that gives colour to hair and skin.
Membrane	A thin elastic tissue covering the surface of certain organs and

lining the cavities of the body.

Metabolism	The sum of all the chemical reactions that take place in living things.
Mucous membrane	Membrane that lines cavities connected with the skin, e.g. the mouth.
Nail bed	The skin underneath the nail.
Nail folds	Three skin folds surrounding the nail.
Nail plate	The hard visible part of the nail structure.
Non-occlusive	That which does not block an opening or openings, such as the pores of the skin.
Nucleic acids	Found in all cells, especially in the nucleus, or control centre, of cells. DNA and RNA are nucleic acids.
Nucleus (plural, nuclei)	The essential part of a cell; the essential agent in growth, metabolism, reproduction and transmission of characteristics of a cell.
Occlusive	Capable of blocking an opening.
Oral	Concerning the mouth.
Orally	By mouth.
Papilla (plural, papillae)	A small nipple-like projection. In the scalp, papillae are cone-like projections which fit into the hair bulbs. They contain minute blood vessels by means of which hair receives nourishment.
Permeability	The quality of being permeable.

Permeable

Capable of allowing the passage of fluids or substances in solution.

PGE1 (prostaglandin E1)

A very important short-lived fatty acid molecule which regulates the activity of the tissues in which it is produced.

pH

Potential of hydrogen. In chemistry, the degrees of acidity or alkalinity of a substance are expressed in pH values.

Photoallergy

See Photosensitivity.

Photosensitivity

Sensitivity to light; a response that occurs when light rays interact with certain chemicals.

Phototoxicity (sun poisoning)

The harmful reaction produced by light energy, particularly by the sun on skin.

Pigment

Any organic colouring matter in the body.

Pimple

A small, often inflamed, protruberance of the skin.

Pituitary gland

An endocrine gland located in the base of the brain. Also known as the hypophysis.

Post-partum

After childbirth.

Precursor

A parent substance from which another substance is made chemically.

Pre-natal

Before birth.

Prostaglandins (PGs)

Highly reactive short-lived molecules. Their main action is that of local messengers which regulate the activity of the tissues in which they are formed.

Proximal

Nearest the point of attachment, centre of the body or point of

	reference. Opposite of distal.
Pruritus	Severe itching. Great irritation of the skin.
Receptor	Group of cells that receive stimuli.
Respiration	Breathing. Inspiration and expiration.
RNA (ribonucleic acid)	The nucleic acid that carries information from the DNA and controls how proteins are made.
Scurvy	A vitamin C deficiency disease.
Sebaceous glands	The oil-secreting glands of the skin.
Seborrhoea	Overactivity of the sebaceous glands. Seborrhoea of the scalp is commonly known as dandruff.
Sebum	The oily secretion of the sebaceous glands.
Sensory	Relating to sensation. Conveying impulses from the sense organs to the brain.
SPF	Sun protection factor.
Stressor	Agent that causes or generates stress.
Subcutaneous	Underneath the skin.
Sudoriferous glands	Sweat-secreting glands of the skin.
Supine	Lying on the back with the face upwards.
Synthesis	The combining of elements or parts to form a whole; the process of building up.
Systemic	Pertaining to the whole body, rather than to one part.

Telogen	Refers to the resting stage of the hair growth cycle.
Tempeh	A sort of cheese made from fermented soya beans.
Thyroid gland	A two-lobed endocrine gland situated in front of the windpipe.
Topical	Pertaining to a definite area; local.
Trichologist	A specialist in the care and treatment of hair.
UV	Ultraviolet. UV rays are invisible rays emitted by very hot bodies, for example, the sun.
Whiteheads	Tiny swollen bumps caused by blockage of openings to the skin's surface. Also known as closed comedones (singular, comedo).

BIBLIOGRAPHY

Airola, Paavo, Ph.D., N.D., *Everywoman's Book. Dr Airola's Practical Guide to Holistic Health*, Phoenix, Arizona, Health Plus Publishers, 1979.

Alive Canadian Journal of Health and Nutrition, No. 63, p. 11, 'Smoking Ages the Skin'.

Angier, Bradford, *Field Guide to Medicinal Wild Plants*, Harrisburg, Pa., USA, Stackpole Books, 1978.

Arndt, Kenneth A., MD, *Manual of Dermatologic Therapeutics with Essentials of Diagnosis* (4th ed.), Boston, Little, Brown and Company, 1989.

Arpel, Adrien, with Ebenstein, Ronnie Sue, *Adrien Arpel's 851 Fast Beauty Fixes and Facts*, New York, G.P. Putnam's Sons, 1985.

Baker, Oleda, and Gale, Bill, 'The Beauty Orgasm', *Cosmopolitan*, pp. 240–243, 250–251, December 1977.

Boyer, Pamela, 'Beauty in the Snow', *Prevention* magazine, pp. 34–35, November 1984.

—— 'Moisturizer Use: Expert Answers', *Prevention* magazine, pp. 51–52, March 1986.

—— 'Bronze, Don't Burn', *Prevention* magazine, pp. 50, 52, 112, May 1986.

Briggs, Colin J., Ph.D., 'Evening Primrose. La Belle de Nuit, the King's Cureall', *Revue Pharmaceutique Canadienne* (Canadian Pharmaceutical Journal), pp. 249–254, May 1986.

Brody, Jane E., *The New York Times' Guide To Personal Health*, New York, Avon Books, 1983.

Burke, Karen E., MD, Ph.D., 'Facial Wrinkles. Prevention and nonsurgical correction' *Postgraduate Medicine*, pp. 207–222, 227, 230, July 1990.

Chaffee, Ellen E., RN, MN, M. Litt, and Lytle, Ivan M., Ph.D., *Basic Physiology and Anatomy* (4th ed.), Philadelphia and Toronto, J.B. Lippincott Company, 1980.

Clarke, B.J. (Ed.), et al., *Self-Medication. A Reference for Health Professionals*, Ottawa, Canada, Canadian Pharmaceutical Association, 1988.

Coninx, Paul, 'Tanning Salons' *Protect Yourself*, pp. 21–27, February 1988.

Connolly, Suzanne M., MD, 'Allergic contact dermatitis. When to suspect and what to do', *Postgraduate Medicine*, Vol. 74, No. 3, pp. 227–235, September 1983.

Davis, Adelle, *Let's Get Well*, New York, Harcourt Brace Jovanovich, Inc., 1965.

—— *Let's Eat Right to Keep Fit*, New York, The New American Library, Inc., 1970.

De Launey, W.E., MB, BS, DDM, FACD, FRACP, and Land, W.A., MB, BS, DDM, FACD, FRACP, *Principles and Practice of Dermatology*, Sydney, Australia, Butterworths, 1978.

Dollery, Eveleen, 'Skin Smarts for Every Decade of a Woman's Life', *Chatelaine* magazine, pp. 68–73, March 1985.

Donsky, Howard, MD, *Beauty Is Skin Deep*, Toronto, Key Porter Books Limited, 1985.

Dvorine, William, MD, *A Dermatologist's Guide to Home Skin Treatment*, Charles Scribner's Sons, 1983.

Elermann, Heinz J., 'The Regulation of Suntan and Sunscreen Products', Washington D.C., Division of Cosmetics Technology, Food and Drug Administration, *Sun Products Documentary Formulary Encyclopedia, Cosmetics & Toiletries*, vol. 98, Allured Publishing Corp., March 1983.

Enriquez, Sanna, B.Sc. (Pharm.), 'Photosensitivity and Sunscreens', *Pharmacy. Continuing Education Highlights*, May–June 1983. Vancouver, Canada, College of Pharmacists of British Columbia.

Erasmus, Udo, *Fats and Oils. The Complete Guide to Fats and Oils in Health and Nutrition*, Vancouver, Canada, Alive Books, 1986.

Feder, Lewis M., MD, and Craig, Jane MacLean, *About Face*, New York, Warner Books, Inc., 1989.

Feltman, John, 'Zinc—The Do-Everything Mineral', *Prevention* magazine, pp. 69–74, November 1979.

Ferri, Elisa, with Siegel, Mary-Ellen, *Finger Tips*, New York, Clarkson N. Potter, Inc., 1988.

Flandermeyer, Kenneth L., MD, *Clear Skin*, Boston, Little, Brown and Company, 1979.

Freifeld, Karen 'Ban That Tan', *Health*, February 1988, pp. 10–11.

Gage, Diane, *Aloe Vera*, Rochester, Vermont, Healing Arts Press, 1988.

Goodman, Thomas, MD. *The Skin Doctor's Skin Doctoring Book*, New York, Sterling Publishing Co. Inc., 1984.

Graham, Judy, *Evening Primrose Oil*, London, England, Thorsons, 1984.

——, and Odent, Dr M., *The Z Factor*, London, Thorsons, 1986.

Green, Barbara, 'The Indoor Tan', *Canadian Consumer*, pp. 28–30, April 1988.

Grieve, Mrs. M., FRHS, *A Modern Herbal* (Vol. I), New York, Dover Publications, Inc., 1971.

Gunnoe, Robert E., MD, 'Diseases of the nails. How to recognize and treat them', *Postgraduate Medicine*, Vol. 74, No. 3, pp. 357–362, September 1983.

Hannifin, Jon M., MD, 'Atopic dermatitis. Special clinical complications', *Postgraduate Medicine*, Vol. 74, No. 3, pp. 188–199, September 1983.

Hanson, Peter G., MD, *The Joy of Stress*, Islington, Ontario, Canada, Hanson Stress Management Organization, 1985.

Harmon, Vera M., RN, MS, and Steele, Shirley M., RN, MA, Ph.D., *Nursing Care of the Skin. A Developmental Approach*, New York, Appleton-Century-Crofts, 1975.

Health League of Canada, 'Lip Tips', *Health League News Digest*, Vol. 5, No. 1, January/February 1986.

—— 'Learn to be Assertive', *Health League News Digest*, Vol. 5, No. 2, March/April 1986.

—— 'Sunburn', *Health League News Digest*, Vol. 5, No. 4, July/August 1986.

Health and Welfare, Minister of, *Dispatch*, No. 44, 1989, Health Protection Branch, Health and Welfare, Canada.

Higgins, Kerry, 'Beauty from the Inside Out', *Mademoiselle*, pp. 79, 165, 167, 168, July 1985.

Horrobin, David F., (Ed.), *Clinical Uses of Essential Fatty Acids*, Montreal, Eden Press Incorporated, 1982.

Houck, Catherine, 'Quick Cures for Holiday Complaints', *New Woman*, p. 138, December 1985.

Jonah, Kathleen, 'The In-Shape Face', *Self* magazine, p. 104, August 1985.

Kaplan, Allen P., MD, 'Chronic Urticaria. Possible causes, suggested treatment alternatives', *Postgraduate Medicine*, Vol. 74, No. 3, pp. 209–221, September 1983.

Kenton, Leslie, *Ageless Ageing*, London, Arrow Books Limited, 1985.

Kingsley, Philip, *The Complete Hair Book*, New York, Grosset & Dunlap, Inc., 1979.

Lam, Anne, B.Sc. Phm., and Grant, David, MD, D.Phil., 'Skin Tanning and Sunscreen Agents — Which product to Use?', *On Continuing Practice*, Vol. 13, No. 2, 1986.

Lappé, Frances Moore, *Diet for a Small Planet*, New York, Ballantine Books, 1971.

LeShan, Lawrence, *How to Meditate*, Wellingborough, England, Turnstone Press Limited, 1983.

Lewis, George M., MD, FACP, *Practical Dermatology* (2nd ed.), Philadelphia and London, W.B. Saunders Company, 1959.

Lubowe, Irwin I., MD, and Huss, Barbara, *A Teen-Age Guide to Healthy Skin and Hair*, New York, E.P. Dutton & Co., Inc., 1965.

McMahon, Judi, and Odell, Zia, *A Year of Beauty & Exercise for the Pregnant Woman*, New York, Lippincott & Crowell, Publishers, 1980.

Maleskey, Gale, 'Vitamins — For External Use Also', *Prevention* magazine, pp. 113–124, July 1984.

Mandell, Jonathan, 'Water. The Fountain of Life', *Reader's Digest*, pp. 11–14, October 1986.

Marieb, Elaine Nicpon, RN, Ph.D., *Essentials of Human Anatomy and Physiology*, Menlo Park, California, Addison-Wesley Publishing Company, Inc., 1984.

Mary Kay Cosmetics, The Beauty Experts at, *The Mary Kay Guide to Beauty*, Reading, Massachusetts, Addison-Wesley, 1983.

Millikan, Larry E., MD, 'Skin and hair disorders', *Postgraduate Medicine*, Vol. 79, No. 5, p. 148, April 1986.

Moi, *Beautiful Nails*, New York, Lippincott & Crowell, Publishers, 1980.

Nazzaro, Dr Ann, Lombard, Dr Donald, and Horrobin, Dr David, *The PMS Solution. Premenstrual Syndrome: The Nutritional Approach*, Montreal, Eden Press, 1985.

Newsweek, 'The Dark Side of the Sun', pp. 60–64, June 9, 1986.

Northorp, Shirley, 'Beautiful Nails', *You* magazine, Summer 1986, Toronto; Family Communications Inc.

Novick, Nelson Lee, MD, *Skin Care for Teens*, New York, Franklin Watts, 1988.

O'Brien, Vicki, *Lifeline*, Vol. 3, No. 3, Vancouver, Canada, Vancouver General Hospital, June 1981.

Ontario Ministry of Health, Canada, 'Good Skin for Life. Make it Yours'.

Passwater, Richard A., Ph.D., *Evening Primrose Oil*, New Canaan, Connecticut, Keats Publishing Inc., 1981.

Pearce, Evelyn, C., SRN, RFN, SCM, MCSP (Teacher's Certificate), *Anatomy and Physiology for Nurses*, London, Faber and Faber Limited, 1956.

Pechter, Kerry, 'Are You Being Skinned Alive?', *Prevention* magazine, pp. 63–65, October 1980.

Pellatt, Sanna G., 'Sunscreens', *Self-Medication. A Reference for Health Professionals*, (Eds. Cheryl Clarke, B.J., et al.), Chapter 4. Ottawa, Canada, Canadian Pharmaceutical Association, 1988.

Perry, Rachel, 'Beauty Basics', *Alive Canadian Journal of Health & Nutrition*, No. 102, p. 17, July 1990.

Peterson, Vicki, *The Natural Food Catalog*, New York, Arco Publishing Company, Inc., 1978.

Phillips, J. Hunter III, MD, Smith, Sharon L., and Storer, James S., MD, 'Hair Loss', *Postgraduate Medicine*, Vol. 79, No. 5, p. 207, April 1986.

Pillsbury, Donald M., MA, D.Sc, (Hon), MD, Shelley, Walter B., MD, Ph.D, and Kligman, Albert M., MD, Ph.D., *Dermatology*,

Philadelphia & London, W.B. Saunders Company, 1956.

Potts, Jerome, F., MD, 'Sunlight, Sunburn, and Sunscreens', *Postgraduate Medicine*, pp. 52–63, June 1990.

Pratt, Jane, *McCall's* magazine, 'How the Sun Affects Your Health', p. 62, August 1985.

Reader's Digest, 'Skin. An Owner's Manual', a complilation, pp. 79–83, July 1986.

Roeder, Giselle, 'Beautifully Alive', *Alive Canadian Journal of Health & Nutrition*, No. 69, p. 17.

——, 'Just Ask Giselle', *Alive Canadian Journal of Health & Nutrition*, No. 31. p. 20.

——, 'Drybrushing Explained', *Alive Canadian Journal of Health & Nutrition*, No. 82, p. 30.

Shaw, Linda, 'Vitamins That Team Up for Clear Skin', *Prevention* magazine, pp. 121–126, December 1979.

Shreeve, Caroline, MD, BS (Lond.), LRCP, MRCS (Eng.), *The Premenstrual Syndrome, The Curse that Can be Cured*, London, England, Thorsons 1983.

—— 'A fresh approach to treating eczema', reprinted from *Modern Medicine*.

Thomas, Clayton L., MD, MPH, *Taber's Cyclopedic Dictionary* (13th ed.), Philadelphia, F.A. Davis Company, 1977.

Torbet, Laura (Ed.), *Helena Rubinstein's Book of the Sun*, New York, Times books, 1979.

Turner, Nancy J., *Food Plants of British Columbia Indians*, Part I/Coastal Peoples, Province of British Columbia, Canada, Ministry of the Provincial Secretary and Government Service Provincial Secretary, 1975.

Weller, Stella, *The Secrets of Stopping Hair Loss*, London, England, Thorsons, 1986.

——, *Pain-free Periods*, London, England, Thorsons, 1986.

——, *Super Natural Immune Power*, London, England, Thorsons, 1989.

——, *Easy Pregnancy with Yoga*, London, England, Thorsons, 1991.

Wesley-Hosford, Zia, *Face Value*, New York, Bantam Books, 1986.

Williams, Roger John, *Nutrition Against Disease*, New York, Pitman Publishing Corp., 1971.

Zizmor, Jonathan, MD, and Foreman, John, *Superhair. The Doctor's Book of Beautiful Hair*, New York, Berkley Publishing Corporation, 1978.
Zizmor, Jonathan, MD, and English, Diane, *Doctor Zizmor's Guide to Clearer Skin*, New York, J.B. Lippincott, 1980.

INDEX